Male Sexual Vitality

*How You Can Benefit from Diet,
Vitamins, Minerals, Herbs, Exercise,
and Other Natural Methods*

Michael T. Murray, N.D.

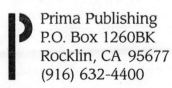

Prima Publishing
P.O. Box 1260BK
Rocklin, CA 95677
(916) 632-4400

Library of Congress Cataloging-in-Publication Data

Murray, Michael T.
   Male sexual vitality / Michael T. Murray.
      p.   cm. — (Getting well naturally series)
   Includes index.
   ISBN 1-55958-428-9
   1. Impotence—Alternative treatment. 2. Infertility—Alternative treatment. 3. Men—Health and hygiene. 4. Herbs—Therapeutic use. 5. Diet therapy. I. Title. II. Series.
   RC889.M87 1994
   616.6'92—dc20   93-29270
                                                   CIP

96 97 98 99 CC 9 8 7 6 5 4 3

Printed in the United States of America

How to Order:

Single copies may be ordered from Prima Publishing, P.O. Box 1260BK, Rocklin, CA 95677; telephone (916) 632-4400. Quantity discounts are also available. On your letterhead, include information concerning the intended use of the books and the number of books you wish to purchase.

Contents

Preface

In many cases we do not realize how important something is until we have lost it. Can you imagine the pain that comes with losing the ability to perform the sexual act, one of life's greatest pleasures? Nearly one out of every four men over the age of 50 knows how it feels to be unable to perform sexually. Even more emotionally painful for many men and their partners is their inability to conceive because the male partner is infertile.

Right or wrong, sex is often at the very center of how a man defines himself. When a man suffers from impotence, premature ejaculation, or is infertile, feelings of inadequacy swell and he no longer feels "like a man." The mere mention of the word *impotence* is enough to send a shiver of fear down the spine of most men. The thought of being unable to perform is simply at direct odds with our image of what is manly.

Throughout history many men have sought immortality. Every man I know does not want to be conquered by the effects of age, yet it is a battle that we all are destined to lose. Yet, should advancing age mean loss of sexual vitality?

Absolutely not. This book provides a detailed program that will enable a man to maintain sexual vitality well into his 80s. Or, if you are a man who has lost sexual vitality, this book can provide answers that may allow you to regain your sexual potency.

This book also provides natural solutions to low sperm counts, prostate disorders, and several other complaints common to men. One of the basic concepts of this book is that, by supplying your body and sexual system with optimal levels of what it needs, it will function optimally. What your body and sexual system need is optimal nutrition and a blood supply that delivers the oxygen and nutrients while removing the waste products. It may sound a bit simple but, for maintaining or attaining health, this is all that it really comes down to in many cases.

The information in this book can change people's lives whether it simply helps a healthy man stay healthy and vital longer, helps a man recover his virility, or helps a couple seeking to create another human life. As significant as the information in this book is, I know that there will always be men who need this information but will never receive it, simply because they may be embarrassed, ashamed, or not willing to admit that they have a problem.

Sexual fulfillment does not have to stop at age 50. If you have not been able to conceive because of a low sperm count or lack of sperm motility, simple nutritional factors may work miracles. There are things that you can do safely, effectively, and naturally to achieve sexual vitality.

Acknowledgments

The major blessings in my life are my family and friends. My love for them truly makes life worth living.

Special appreciation: to my wife, Gina, for being the answer to so many of my dreams; to my parents, Cliff and Patty Murray, and my grandmother, Pauline Shier, for a strong foundation and a lifetime of good memories; to Bob and Kathy Bunton for their love and acceptance; to Ben Dominitz and everyone at Prima for their commitment and support of my work; to Terry Lemerond and everyone at Enzymatic Therapy for all their friendship and support over the years; to Joseph Pizzorno and the students and faculty at Bastyr College, who have given me encouragement and support; and finally, I am eternally grateful to all the researchers, physicians, and scientists who over the years have strived to better understand the use of natural medicines. Without their work, this series would not exist, and medical progress would halt.

Michael T. Murray, N.D.
August 1993

Before You Read On

- Do not self-diagnose. Proper medical care is critical to good health. If you have symptoms suggestive of an illness, please consult a physician—preferably, a naturopath, holistic physician or osteopath, chiropractor, or other natural health care specialist.
- If you are currently taking a prescription medication, you absolutely must consult your doctor before discontinuing it.
- If you wish to try the natural approach, discuss it with your physician. Since he or she is most likely unaware of the natural alternatives available, you may need to do some educating. Bring this book along with you to the doctor's office. The natural alternatives being recommended are based upon published studies in medical journals. Key references are provided if your physician wants additional information.
- Remember, although many natural alternatives, such as nutritional supplements and plant-based medicines, are effective on their own, they work even better if they are part of a comprehensive natural treatment plan that focuses on diet and lifestyle.

1 ⚘

The Male Sexual System

The male sexual system is composed of the testes, genital ducts, accessory glands, and penis. Figure 1.1 illustrates the various components of the male reproductive system. Figure 1.2 shows in detail the structure of the testes (testicles) and epididymis.

Testes

The testes lie within the scrotal sac. The scrotal sac performs an important role: It maintains the testes at a temperature about 2 degrees Celsius below the temperature of the internal organs, so sperm formation can occur. Nature placed the testicles outside the body and equipped them with a special set of muscles that draw them close to the body when they get too cold and drop them farther away when the temperature rises too high. In addition to functioning as the location for sperm formation, the testes are responsible for hormonal output.

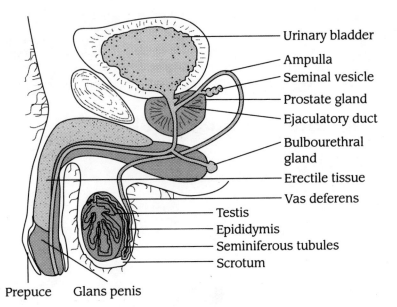

Urinary bladder
Ampulla
Seminal vesicle
Prostate gland
Ejaculatory duct
Bulbourethral gland
Erectile tissue
Vas deferens
Testis
Epididymis
Seminiferous tubules
Scrotum
Prepuce   Glans penis

Figure 1.1 The male reproductive system

Each testis is surrounded by a thick, sturdy capsule of connective tissue known as the tunica albuginea, which serves as a protective shield for this somewhat exposed organ. Inside the testis there are about 250 compartments known as testicular lobules. Each lobule is composed of from one to four tubules called seminiferous tubules. Each tubule would be from 1½ to 2 feet long if straightened out.

It is inside the seminiferous tubule that sperm formation takes place with the aid of special nutrient-providing cells called Sertoli cells. Sertoli cells are known to have at least four main functions: (1) support, protection, and nutritional regulation of the developing sperm; (2) the breakdown of cellular debris cast off by developing sperm; (3) the secretion of a fluid that is utilized for sperm transport; and (4) the excretion of estrogen and a binding protein for testosterone.

The seminiferous tubules are immersed in a web of blood and lymphatic vessels, loose connective tissue, nerves,

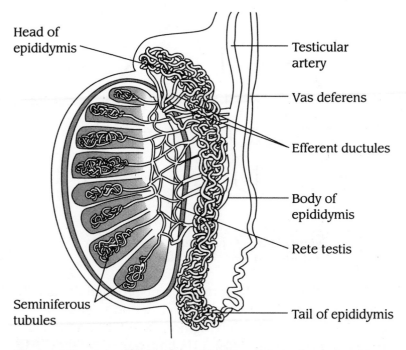

Head of epididymis

Testicular artery

Vas deferens

Efferent ductules

Body of epididymis

Rete testis

Seminiferous tubules

Tail of epididymis

Figure 1.2 Internal structure of the testicle and relationship of the testicle to the epididymis

and special cells known as Leydig cells. These cells are responsible for the production and secretion of testosterone. Leydig cells are almost nonexistent in the testes during childhood, but they are numerous and quite active in the newborn male infant and also in the adult male after puberty. After birth and at puberty, the testes secrete relatively large quantities of testosterone. Figure 1.3 shows rates of testosterone secretion at different ages.

Spermatogenesis

Fully developed sperm (spermatozoa) are produced via a process known as spermatogenesis. Figure 1.4 shows the

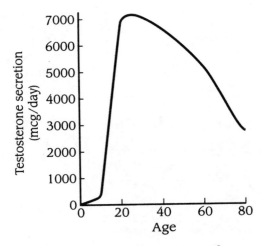

Figure 1.3 Approximate rates of testosterone secretion at different ages

structure of a normal sperm. Sperm production usually begins around puberty, as a result of the release of the pituitary hormones leutinizing hormone (LH) and follicle-stimulating hormone (FSH). LH stimulates Leydig cells to produce testosterone; FSH stimulates Sertoli cells to produce sperm. Although not as well known as testosterone, both LH and FSH are critical to sperm formation.

Functions of Testosterone

In general, testosterone is the hormone responsible for the distinguishing characteristics of the masculine body. During fetal development, testosterone leads to the development of the male sexual apparatus: scrotum, penis, testes, prostate gland, and seminal vesicles. At the same time, testosterone suppresses the formation of female genital organs. Shortly after birth, the testosterone level drops and remains quite low until puberty.

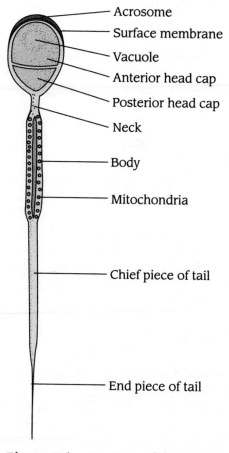

Figure 1.4 Structure of the human sperm

After puberty and before the age of 20, testosterone causes the penis, scrotum, and testes to enlarge about eightfold. At this stage, testosterone leads to the development of male secondary sexual characteristics, including distribution of body hair, lower voice, thickness of the skin, and increased muscular development.

The Genital Ducts

The genital ducts' function is to transport out of the body the sperm produced in the testis. The first passageway is the epididymis, one long, highly tortuous tube about 20 feet in length. As the sperm make the passage through the epididymis, they begin to mature. After being in the epididymis for 18 to 24 hours, the sperm become more motile. (Inhibitory fluids secreted by the epididymis prevent full motility until after ejaculation.)

From the epididymis, the sperm travel up through the vas deferens, also called the ductus deferens, a straight tube with thick walls. Before the vas penetrates the prostate, it dilates and forms a region known as the ampulla. At the final portion of the ampulla, the seminal vesicles join it to form a duct. Upon entering the prostate, before it empties into the urethra, the duct is called the ejaculatory duct.

Accessory Glands

The male accessory sex glands are the seminal vesicles, prostate, and bulbourethral glands.

It was thought for a long time that sperm were stored in the seminal vesicles, hence their name. We now know that sperm are not stored in these glands. The primary function of the seminal vesicles is the secretion of a fluid that provides nutrients to sperm and increases sperm motility. Substances secreted by the seminal vesicles include fructose, which nourishes the sperm, and large quantities of prostaglandins and fibrinogen. Prostaglandins are hormonelike substances produced from essential fatty acids. Prostaglandins are thought to aid fertilization by reacting with the mucus of the vagina and cervix to make them more hospitable to sperm. Possibly, prostaglandins cause contractions in the uterus and fallopian tubes to move the sperm toward the ovaries. The fibrinogen combines with prostatic secretions to form a weak coagulate that holds the semen together after ejaculation, allowing it to find the deeper regions of the vagina. The coagulate also limits sperm motility. Because the coagulate dissolves 15 to 20 minutes after ejaculation, however, the sperm soon become highly motile.

About 60% of the volume of semen is composed of secretions from the seminal vesicles. The remainder of the semen (30% of the total volume) is composed of prostatic fluid and secretions from the vas deferens. Sperm and fluid compose 10% of total volume.

The prostate is a single, doughnut-shaped gland about the size of a walnut. It lies below the bladder and surrounds the urethra. The prostate secretes a thin, milky, alkaline fluid that lubricates the urethra to prevent infection. In addition, the fluid increases sperm motility. The alkaline nature of the prostatic secretion is extremely important to successful fertilization of the egg, because the fluid of the vas deferens as well as the vaginal secretions are relatively acidic. Sperm do not become optimally mobile until the pH of the surrounding fluids rises to 6 to 6.5. Consequently, the prostatic fluid plays an important role in promoting sperm motility by neutralizing the acid and raising the pH of semen to 7.5.

The bulbourethral glands are pea-sized formations located below the prostate and around the urethra. The bulbourethral glands produce a thin, milky secretion that lubricates the urethra and prepares the urethra for the transport of the semen.

The Penis

The penis consists primarily of erectile tissue, the urethra, and blood vessels, all surrounded externally by skin. The penis is divided into two distinct sections, the shaft and the head (glans penis). The glans is the most important source of nerve impulses that signal the sexual response. The shaft of the penis contains erectile tissue that is housed in three cylindrical masses. Two, the corpus cavernosum, are located around central arteries and one, the corpus spongiosum, surrounds the urethra. Figure 1.5 shows the structure of the penis.

Erection is the result of dilation of the arteries in the penis, combined with the filling of the erectile tissue. In simple terms, an erection requires that the volume of blood entering the penis exceed the volume leaving it. The erectile tissue is really nothing more than large, cavernous, blood storage compartments. These compartments are normally relatively empty, but they become tremendously dilated when arterial blood flows rapidly into them under pressure and the outflow is partially occluded. The erectile tissue is surrounded by a strong membrane composed of hard fibers. The membrane greatly increases the pressure within the ballooning erectile tissue; therefore, the penis becomes hard and elongated.

The Stages of the Male Sexual Act

The male sexual act is initiated in most instances by an interplay of psychic and physical stimulation. Simply

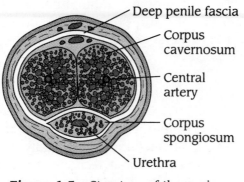

Figure 1.5 Structure of the penis

thinking sexual thoughts or dreaming that the act of sexual intercourse is taking place can lead to an erection and even ejaculation. Most men at some point in their sexual development (usually their teen years) experience nocturnal emissions during dreams. (Such dreams are usually called wet dreams.)

Although psychic factors obviously contribute to the male sexual response, it is interesting to note that they are not absolutely necessary to the performance of the male sexual act. Due to an inherent reflex mechanism, appropriate genital stimulation can lead to erection and ejaculation without psychic stimuli. For example, some individuals with spinal cord damage that prevents the transmission of nerve impulses from the brain are still capable of achieving erection and ejaculation.

So, either psychic or physical stimulation can initiate the sexual act. Physical stimulation to sensitive tissue, primarily the glans penis, but also the entire pubic region, sends nerve impulses to the sacral portion of the spinal cord, causing a reflex impulse to the penis. This leads to dilation of the arteries and to blood filling the erectile tissue. In addition, these same nerve impulses cause the bulbourethral glands to secrete mucus that lubricates the urethra and aids intercourse.

The initial nerve stimulus from the spinal cord during the sexual act is controlled by the parasympathetic nervous system. The parasympathetic system controls bodily functions such as digestion, breathing, and heart rate during periods of rest, relaxation, visualization, meditation, and sleep. In contrast, the sympathetic nervous system is designed to protect against immediate danger and is responsible for the so-called fight or flight reaction. Although the parasympathetic nervous system is responsible for erection and lubrication, the sympathetic nervous system controls emission and ejaculation.

Emission and ejaculation are the culmination of the male sexual act. When sexual stimulation becomes extremely intense, the reflex centers of the spinal cord begin to emit sympathetic nerve impulses to initiate emission, the fore-runner of ejaculation.

Emission begins with contraction of the vas deferens, the tubule that transports the sperm from the epididymis to the prostate. Contraction of the vas deferens leads to the expulsion of sperm into the ejaculatory duct and urethra. Then, contractions of the prostate and seminal vesicles expel prostatic and seminal fluid into the ejaculatory duct, thus forcing the sperm into the urethra. All these fluids, along with the secretions of the bulbourethral glands, mix in the internal urethra to form semen.

The filling of the urethra elicits sensory nerve impulses that further excite rhythmic contractions of the internal organs and also cause the rhythmic contraction of the erectile tissues. Together, these contractions lead to a tremendous increase in pressure, which ejaculates the semen from the urethra. Simultaneously, the pelvic muscles and even the muscles of the abdomen cause thrusting movements of the pelvis and penis, which also help propel the semen.

The entire process of emission and ejaculation is known as the male orgasm. Within 1 or 2 minutes after ejaculation, male sexual excitement disappears almost entirely and erection disappears.

Chapter Summary

The male sexual system is composed of the testes, genital ducts, accessory glands, and penis. The reproductive function of this system is to deliver viable sperm to the vagina.

2

Erectile Dysfunction

The term *impotence* has traditionally been used to signify the inability of a male to attain and maintain erection of the penis sufficient to permit satisfactory sexual intercourse. A more precise term than *impotence,* in most circumstances, is *erectile dysfunction.* This term differentiates difficulty with erection from loss of libido, premature ejaculation, or inability to achieve orgasm.[1]

An estimated 10 to 20 million men suffer from erectile dysfunction. This number is expected to increase dramatically as the median age of the population increases. Currently, erectile dysfunction is thought to affect over 25% of men over the age of 50.[1,2]

Although the frequency of erectile dysfunction increases with age, it must be stressed that aging itself is not a cause of impotence. Although the amount and force of the ejaculate as well as the need to ejaculate decrease with age, the capacity for erection remains. Men are capable of retaining their sexual virility well into their 80s.

Erectile dysfunction can be due to organic or psychogenic (mental or emotional) factors. In the overwhelming majority of cases, the cause is organic—that is, it is due to some physiological reason. In fact, in men over the age of 50, organic causes are responsible for over 90% of all cases of erectile dysfunction.[3] In the past, an "impotent" man who was able to have nighttime or early-morning erections was thought to have a psychogenic problem. This is no longer the case; factors other than mental or emotional conflict may be involved.[2]

Causes of Erectile Dysfunction

Figure 2.1 lists the major causes of erectile dysfunction. This chapter will discuss a few of the most significant.

Organic (85%)
Vascular insufficiency
  Atherosclerosis
  Insufficiency resulting
    from pelvic surgery, pelvic
    trauma, or venous shunting
  Venous leakage

Drugs
  Antihistamines
  Antihypertensives
  Anticholinergics
  Antidepressants
  Antipsychotics
  Tranquilizers
  Others

Alcohol and tobacco

Endocrine disorders
  Diabetes
  Hypothyroidism

  Low levels of male sex
    hormones
  Elevated prolactin level
  High estrogen level

*Diseases or trauma to male
sexual organs*
  Diseases of the penis
  Prostate disorders

Neurological diseases
  Diseases resulting in
    pelvic trauma or surgery
  Multiple sclerosis

Psychological (10%)
Psychiatric illness
  Stress
  Performance anxiety
  Depression

Unknown (5%)

Figure 2.1   Causes of erectile dysfunction

Medical history

Physical examination

Laboratory studies
   Complete blood count and urinalysis
   Biochemical profile
   Glucose tolerance test
   Serum hormone levels

Psychological evaluation
   Minnesota Multiphasic Personality Inventory

Nocturnal penile monitoring

Neurological examination

Vascular examination

Figure 2.2   Means used to evaluate erectile dysfunction

Since correction of any underlying organic factor is the first step in restoring sexual function, proper diagnosis is critical. Figure 2.2 lists some of the procedures used to attain a diagnosis. A thorough history and physical exam are often all that are needed for diagnosis. In some cases, noninvasive tests can diagnose the cause of erectile dysfunction. These tests are best performed or supervised by a urologist.

Atherosclerosis

By far the most common cause of erectile dysfunction is vascular disease. Atherosclerosis of the penile artery is the primary cause in nearly half the men over the age of 50 who suffer from erectile dysfunction.[1] Atherosclerosis is the hardening of artery walls, and it is due to a buildup of plaque containing cholesterol, fatty material, and cellular debris. Atherosclerosis and its complications are the major causes of death in the United States. Heart disease, one result of atherosclerosis, accounts for 36% of all deaths in the United States; it is the number one killer of Americans. Stroke, another complication of atherosclerosis, is the third most common cause of death in the United States. Altogether, atherosclerosis is responsible for at least 43% of all U.S. deaths. Erectile dysfunction due to atherosclerosis has been shown to be a harbinger of heart attack or stroke.[3] The process of atherosclerosis occurs throughout the body, not just in the arteries supplying the heart or penis. Compared to individuals without coronary disease, patients with diseased coronary arteries are much more likely to have erectile dysfunction. If erectile dysfunction is due to vascular insufficiency, the patient must take measures to reduce cardiovascular risk. These measures should focus on lowering cholesterol and triglyceride levels, decreasing blood pressure, reducing obesity, eliminating smoking, and increasing exercise.

The diagnosis of erectile dysfunction due to atherosclerosis can be made with ultrasound techniques. A patient who receives such a diagnosis should also have his blood cholesterol and triglyceride levels checked. (Table 2.1 shows recommended levels.) A total cholesterol level above 200 milligrams per deciliter is a strong indication that atherosclerosis may be responsible for decreased blood flow.

When physicians suspect that erectile dysfunction is due to a vascular problem, they may inject papaverine into the penis during the clinical evaluation. Papaverine is a drug that dilates arteries, causing them to deliver more blood to erectile tissues. If erectile dysfunction is due to arterial insufficiency, the penis will become erect and the erection will be sustained. If the erection cannot be maintained, venous leakage is the probable cause of the dysfunction. Venous leakage is much more difficult to treat than insufficient blood flow; venous leakage may require surgery.

Reversing Atherosclerosis The dietary recommendations in Chapter 6 will prevent as well as reverse (yes, *reverse*) atherosclerosis. The ability of diet to protect against

Table 2.1   Recommended Blood Cholesterol
and Triglyceride Levels

Blood Component	Recommended Level
Total cholesterol	Less than 200 mg/dL
LDL cholesterol	Less than 130 mg/dL
HDL cholesterol	Greater than 35 mg/dL
Triglycerides	50 to 150 mg/dL

atherosclerosis is well accepted, but more and more evidence supports the view that diet and lifestyle can dramatically reverse the blocking of arteries. The dietary guidelines provided in Chapter 6 are quite similar to those that reversed atherosclerosis in the now-famous Lifestyle Heart Trial conducted by Dr. Dean Ornish.[4]

In the Lifestyle Heart Trial, subjects with heart disease were placed into one of two groups: a control group and an experimental group. Those in the control group received regular medical care and followed the diet prescribed by the American Heart Association. The experimental group ate a lowfat vegetarian diet for at least one year. The diet included fruits, vegetables, grains, legumes, and soybean products. These subjects were allowed to consume as many calories as they wished. No animal products were allowed except egg white and 1 cup per day of nonfat milk or yogurt. The diet contained approximately 10% fat; 15% to 20% protein; and 70% to 75% carbohydrate, which was predominantly complex carbohydrate from whole grains, legumes, and vegetables.

The experimental group practiced stress reduction techniques—such as breathing, stretching, and imagery exercises, and meditation—for an hour each day. In addition, this group performed physical exercise at least 3 hours per week. At the end of the year, the subjects in the experimental group showed significant overall regression of atherosclerosis of the coronary blood vessels. In contrast, subjects in the control group actually showed progression of their disease. In other words, the group following standard medical treatment actually got worse. As Ornish stated: "This finding suggests that conventional recommendations for patients with coronary heart disease (such as a 30% fat diet) are not sufficient to bring about regression in many patients."

As well as following an effective diet and maintaining a healthful lifestyle, following the nutritional supplementation recommendations given in Chapter 7 is important. As you will learn, several of the antioxidant nutrients (such as vitamins C and E, beta-carotene, and selenium) can offer significant protection against atherosclerosis.

Another means of lowering cholesterol is niacin. Niacin, or vitamin B3, has long been used for this purpose. In fact, the National Cholesterol Education Program recommended niacin as the first "drug" to use to reduce cholesterol.[5] Niacin was the only substance associated with decreased mortality in the famed Coronary Drug Project.[6] Niacin can cause problems, however. The dose required (1 gram, three times per day) often results in flushing of the skin, stomach irritation, ulcers, liver damage, fatigue, and other side effects. Because of these side effects, a physician should supervise most niacin therapy for lowering cholesterol.

The safest form of niacin available is inositol hexaniacinate. It is composed of one molecule of inositol (an unofficial B vitamin) and six molecules of niacin. Inositol hexaniacinate has been used in Europe for over 30 years to lower cholesterol and improve blood flow. Compared to niacin, inositol hexaniacinate yields slightly better results than standard niacin, and the body tolerates it better. It causes less flushing and, more important, causes fewer long-term side effects.[7-9] Inositol hexaniacinate is available at health food stores. A dosage effective for lowering cholesterol levels is 1,000 to 3,000 milligrams per day.

In the case of erectile dysfunction, inositol hexaniacinate may offer an additional benefit: improved blood flow. In fact,

Europeans use it more for its ability to improve the circulation than for its cholesterol-lowering effects.

Prescription Medications

There is a long list of prescription medications that can interfere with sexual function. If you are taking a medication of any sort and are impotent, consult your physician, pharmacist, or the book *Physicians' Desk Reference* to determine if the drug could be responsible. If it is, work with your physician to get off the medication. For most common health conditions, natural measures can be used to produce safer and better clinical results. For more information, consult *The Encyclopedia of Natural Medicine* (by Michael T. Murray and Joseph E. Pizzorno, Prima Publishing, Rocklin, California, 1992).

The most common drugs that cause erectile dysfunction are those designed to lower blood pressure (antihypertensive drugs). These include diuretics, beta-blockers, calcium channel-blockers, and angiotensin-converting enzyme inhibitors. In most instances these drugs are prescribed needlessly. Virtually every medical authority (be it a textbook, organization, journal, or what have you)—including the Joint National Committee on Detection, Evaluation and Treatment of High Blood Pressure—has recommended that nondrug therapies be used in the treatment of borderline to moderate hypertension (a blood pressure less than 150/105 millimeters of mercury). The use of antihypertensives results in no benefit for most patients and involves significant risks besides erectile dysfunction. The two most definitive trials of blood pressure–lowering drugs (the Australian and Medical Research Council trials), as well as five other large trials (including the famous Multiple Risk Factor Intervention Trial), showed that the drugs did not protect against heart disease in patients with borderline to moderate hypertension.[10]

Alcohol and Tobacco

In addition to increasing the risk for atherosclerosis, long-term alcohol consumption or tobacco use is often a big contributor to erectile dynsfunction. Alcohol can produce acute episodes of impotence as well as impotence due to testicular shrinkage. Smoking just two cigarettes has been shown to inhibit penile erection produced by injection of a low dose of papaverine.[3]

Endocrine Disorders

A variety of endocrine and hormonal disorders can lead to erectile dysfunction. The most common of these is diabetes. Compared to nondiabetics, diabetics are at higher risk for atherosclerosis and nerve damage, both of which can cause impotence. If you are a diabetic, please consult *Diabetes and Hypoglycemia* (by Michael T. Murray, Prima Publishing, Rocklin, California, 1994), another book in the Getting Well Naturally series.

Other relatively common results of endocrine disorders that cause erectile dysfunction include excess prolactin, low levels of testosterone (hypogonadism), and hypothyroidism. Blood measurements are required to determine prolactin and testosterone levels. If the level of prolactin is high, follow the recommendations given in Chapter 4, in the section called "The Natural Approach to BPH and Prostatitis." If the testosterone level is slightly low, follow the recommendations given in Chapter 3, in the section called "The Natural Approach to Oligospermia and Azoospermia." In addition, try taking *Panax ginseng* (also called Korean ginseng or Chinese ginseng), as discussed in Chapter 8. If the level of testosterone is very low, however, a physician may have to prescribe the hormone for you.

Hypothyroidism

Since the hormones of the thyroid gland regulate metabolism in every cell of the body, a deficiency of thyroid hormones can affect virtually all body functions. In the adult, hypothyroidism ranges from extremely mild deficiency states (subclinical hypothyroidism) that are barely detectable, to severe deficiency states (myxedema) that are life threatening.

Much controversy surrounds the diagnosis of hypothyroidism. Before the components of blood could be measured with accuracy, diagnosis of hypothyroidism was based on basal body temperature (the temperature of the body at rest) and Achilles tendon reflex time (hypothyroidism slows reflexes). With the advent of sophisticated laboratory measurement of thyroid hormones in the blood, these tests of thyroid function fell by the wayside. However, it is now known that blood tests are not sensitive enough to diagnose mild forms of hypothyroidism. Because mild hypothyroidism is the most common form, the majority of people with hypothyroidism are going undiagnosed.

The basal body temperature is perhaps the most sensitive indicator of thyroid function. A simple method for taking your basal body temperature follows.

Taking Your Basal Body Temperature   Your body temperature reflects your metabolic rate, which is largely determined by hormones secreted by the thyroid gland. Therefore, by simply knowing your basal body temperature, you and your physician can get an idea of how well your thyroid gland is functioning. All you need is a thermometer.

Procedure

Menstruating women must perform the test on the second, third, and fourth days of menstruation. Men and postmenopausal women can perform the test, upon waking, at any time of the month.

1. Shake the thermometer so the mercury is below 95 degrees Fahrenheit. Place the thermometer by your bed before going to sleep at night.
2. On waking, place the thermometer in your armpit for a full 10 minutes. Move as little as possible. Lie still and rest with your eyes closed. Do not get up until the 10-minute test is completed.
3. After 10 minutes, read and record the temperature and date.
4. Record the temperature for at least three mornings (preferably at the same time of day) and give the information to your physician.

Interpreting Basal Body Temperature   Your basal body temperature should be between 97.6 and 98.2 degrees Fahrenheit. Low basal body temperatures are quite common and may reflect hypothyroidism. Other common signs and symptoms of hypothyroidism are depression, difficulty in losing weight, dry skin, headaches, lethargy or fatigue, loss of libido, menstrual problems, recurrent infections, constipation, and sensitivity to cold.

High basal body temperatures (above 98.6 degrees) are less common than low temperatures, but they may be evidence of hyperthyroidism. Common signs and symptoms of hyperthyroidism include bulging eyeballs, fast pulse, hyperactivity, inability to gain weight, insomnia, irritability, menstrual problems, and nervousness.

Correcting Hypothyroidism   The medical treatment of hypothyroidism, in all but the mildest form of the disease, involves the use of desiccated thyroid or synthetic thyroid hormone. Although synthetic hormones have become popular, many physicians (particularly naturopathic physicians) prefer the use of desiccated natural thyroid, complete with all thyroid hormones. At this time, it appears that thyroid hormone replacement is necessary for the majority of people with hypothyroidism.

Thyroxine is one of the hormones the thyroid gland secretes. The primary purpose of this hormone is to increase the rate of cell metabolism. The Food and Drug Administration requires the thyroid extracts sold in health food stores to be thyroxine-free according to FDA standards. However, it is nearly impossible to remove all the hormone from the gland. In other words, think of health food–store thyroid preparations as mild forms of desiccated natural thyroid. If you have mild hypothyroidism, such a preparation may provide the support you need to overcome your thyroid problem.

The potency and amount of nutrients in a nonprescription thyroid preparation vary from one manufacturer to the next. Therefore, in regard to dosage, follow the manufacturer's recommendations, as provided on the product label. Use your basal body temperature to determine the effectiveness of the product.

Like hormone therapy, diet plays an important role in correcting hypothyroidism. The goal of the dietary approach is to ensure the intake of the nutrients that are required for the manufacture of thyroid hormones. These nutrients include iodine, zinc, vitamin A, and copper. A deficiency of these, in particular, can result in hypothyroidism.

Adequate intake of iodine is especially important because a deficiency of iodine causes the cells of the thyroid gland to enlarge. Enlargement of the thyroid gland, when it is caused by lack of iodine, is called goiter. Goiter affects over 200 million people the world over. In all but 4% of cases, it is caused by iodine deficiency. Iodine deficiency is now quite rare in the United States and other industrialized countries, because of the addition of iodine to table salt. (Adding iodine to table salt began in Michigan, where in 1924 the goiter rate was an incredible 47%.)

These days, few Americans are iodine deficient. Nevertheless, the rate of goiter is still relatively high (5% to 6%) in certain high-risk areas. Goiter sufferers in these areas are probably eating certain foods that block iodine utilization. These foods, called goitrogens, include turnips, cabbage, mustard, cassava root, soybeans, peanuts, pine nuts, and millet. The cooking process usually inactivates goitrogens.

The recommended dietary allowance (RDA) of iodine for adults is quite small, 150 micrograms. Seafoods— including seaweeds like kelp, clams, lobsters, oysters, sardines, and other saltwater fish—are nature's richest sources of iodine. However, the majority of iodine Americans consume is from iodized salt—70 micrograms of iodine per gram of iodized salt. (Sea salt has little iodine.) The average intake of iodine in the United States is estimated to be over 600 micrograms per day per person.

Too much iodine can actually inhibit thyroid gland synthesis. For this reason and because the only function of iodine in the body is in thyroid hormone synthesis, daily intake of iodine through dietary sources and supplementation should not exceed 1 milligram (1,000 micrograms) per day per person for any length of time.

Diseases or Trauma of Male Sexual Organs

Diseases of the penis, such as Peyronie's disease, and prostate disorders are among the most common problems that cause erectile dysfunction. Chapter 4 will focus on prostate disorders, so this section will be devoted to Peyronie's disease.

Peyronie's disease is a disorder in which part of the sheath of fibrous connective tissue within the penis thickens. As a result, the penis bends during erection. Intercourse is often difficult and quite painful. Although Peyronie's disease sometimes improves without treatment, my recommendation to men with Peyronie's disease is to take a concentrated extract of *Centella asiatica* along with the enzyme bromelain.

Centella contains compounds that can normalize connective tissue and possibly reverse Peyronie's disease. The only commercial source of the extract that I know of that contains the proper concentration of active compounds (triterpenic acids) is Cellu-Var, a product of Enzymatic Therapy. Take 2 capsules, twice daily.

Bromelain is the protein-digesting enzyme of pineapple. It prevents the deposition of fibrin. Deposition of fibrin is thought to be responsible for the thickening of the fibrous connective tissue in the penis. If you have Peyronie's disease, take 750 milligrams of bromelain, three times daily, on an empty stomach. Taking the enzyme 20 minutes before meals works well.

Several men for whom I have prescribed Cellu-Var and bromelain have experienced substantial improvement within the first two weeks of therapy. Give the program at least six weeks to show results.

Medical Treatment of Erectile Dysfunction

The standard medical treatment of erectile dysfunction ranges from relatively noninvasive measures to the placement of prosthetic devices within the penis. The therapeutic options include:

Psychotherapy
Vacuum constrictive devices
Intercavernosal injection
Medications
Penile prosthesis

Psychotherapy

Psychological therapies for impotence are useful in some cases, but keep in mind that in men over the age of 50, psychological factors are rarely the cause of erectile dysfunction. Nonetheless, impotence can lead to psychological disturbances. Even in cases of clear-cut organic erectile dysfunction, repeated inability to attain or sustain an erection leads men to frustration, anxiety, and anticipation of failure. Learning stress reduction techniques (relaxation exercises, biofeedback, and deep-breathing exercises, for example) may help reduce anxiety. In addition, psychological treatment may be especially beneficial for patients who are depressed.

Vacuum Constrictive Devices

Vacuum constrictive devices literally pump blood into the erectile tissue. Most of these devices consist of a vacuum chamber, a pump, connector tubing, and penile constrictor bands. The vacuum chamber is large enough to fit over the erect penis. The connector tube runs to the pump from a small opening at the closed end of the container. An elastic constrictor band is placed around the base of the chamber. Water-soluble lubricant is applied to the open end of the cylinder and to the entire penis. The chamber is placed over the flaccid penis, and an airtight seal is obtained.

The pump (some are battery-operated) creates a vacuum in the chamber. The negative pressure draws blood into the penis, to produce an erectionlike state. The constrictor band is then guided from the vacuum chamber onto the base of the penis. The erection is maintained because the blood is trapped in the penis.

Although manufacturers and many physicians state that vacuum devices have revolutionized the management of erectile dysfunction, patient acceptance does not reflect this enthusiasm. Vacuum constrictive devices are generally effective and are extremely safe, but for some reason a significant numer of patients quit using them. The reason may be that the devices are somewhat uncomfortable, cumbersome, and difficult to use; it takes patience and persistence to master the process. Most vacuum devices require both hands or the assistance of the sexual partner. Patients may quit using these devices because they may impair ejaculation and cause discomfort. Patients and partners complain about the lack of spontaneity that results from the use of vacuum devices. Despite these short-comings, vacuum constrictive devices have been used successfully by many men with erectile dysfunction.[11]

Intercavernosal Self-Injection

Injection of drugs that dilate the penile arteries is a popular method of treatment of erectile dysfunction due to vascular insufficiency. The most common drugs used include papaverine, prostaglandin E1, and phentolamine. Although these drugs have not received FDA approval for treating erectile dysfunction, they are widely used—either singly or in combination.[1,3]

The patient injects the medication into his penis when he wants to have intercourse. The major side effects of this therapy are priapism (inappropriately persistent erections that are often quite painful), bruising, urethral bleeding, scar formation, and low blood pressure. Like the vacuum devices, there is a high rate of patient dropout with self-injection.

Prescription Medications to Improve Erectile Function

Several drugs have been reported to improve erectile function. Testosterone is useful in cases of low testosterone. Bromocriptine, a drug that blocks prolactin secretion by the pituitary, is useful in normalizing prolactin levels and improving sexual function in men with elevated prolactin levels.[3]

The FDA approves only one medicine for impotence: yohimbine, an alkaloid isolated from the bark of the yohimbe tree (*Pausinystalia johimbe*), native to tropical West Africa. Yohimbine hydrochloride increases libido, but its primary action is to increase blood flow to erectile tissue. Contrary to a popular misconception, yohimbine has no effect on the testosterone level.

When used alone, yohimbine is successful in 34% to 43% of cases.[12,13] If combined with strychnine and testosterone, it is even more effective. However, side effects often make yohimbine difficult to utilize. Yohimbine can induce anxiety, panic attacks, and hallucinations. Other side effects include elevation of blood pressure and heart rate, dizziness, headache, and skin flushing. Yohimbine should not be used by those with kidney disease or psychological problems or by women.

Penile Prostheses

The "gold standard" for the treatment of erectile dysfunction is the surgical insertion of a penile prosthesis.[1,11] Implantation of such a device is the "treatment of choice in most cases of complete impotence."[11] Three forms are available: semirigid, malleable, and inflatable. The effectiveness, complications, and acceptability vary according to type. The main problems of all three are mechanical failure, infection, erosion of the connective tissue, and irreversible damage to erectile tissue.

Obviously, insertion of a penile prosthesis should be viewed not as the first step in the treatment of erectile dysfunction, but rather the very last step, after all other attempts have proved futile.

The Natural Approach to Erectile Dysfunction

Although potency is largely dependent upon adequate male sex hormones, adequate sensory stimulation, and adequate blood supply to the erectile tissues, all these factors are dependent upon adequate nutrition. Therefore, it can be concluded that nutrition plays a major role in determining virility.

The diet and nutritional supplementation program in Chapters 6 and 7 provides the fuel men need to function at their best. A diet rich in whole foods—particularly vegetables, fruits, whole grains, and legumes—is extremely important. Adequate protein is also a must, although it is better to get high-quality protein from fish, chicken, turkey, and lean cuts of beef (preferably hormone-free) than from fat-filled sources such as hamburgers, roasts, and pork.

Specific foods often recommended to enhance virility include liver, oysters, nuts, seeds, and legumes. All these foods are good sources of zinc. Zinc is perhaps the most important nutrient for sexual function. Zinc is concentrated in semen, and frequent ejaculation can greatly diminish zinc in the body. If a zinc deficiency exists, the body appears to respond by reducing sexual drive as a mechanism by which to hold on to this important trace mineral.

Other key nutrients for sexual function include essential fatty acids, vitamin A, vitamin B6, and vitamin E. A high-potency multiple vitamin and mineral formula ensures adequate intake of these nutrients, as well as others important in health and sexual function.

In addition to nutrition, the natural approach to erectile dysfunction utilizes exercise and plant-based medicines.

Exercise

The immediate effect of exercise is stress on the body. However, with a regular exercise program, the body adapts; it becomes stronger, functions more efficiently, and has greater endurance. Exercise is a vital component of health, especially sexual health.

The entire body benefits from regular exercise, largely as a result of improved cardiovascular and respiratory function. Simply stated, exercise enhances the transport of oxygen and nutrients into cells. At the same time, exercise enhances the transport of carbon dioxide and waste products from the tissues of the body to the bloodstream and, ultimately, to eliminative organs.

Regular exercise is particularly important in reducing the risk of heart disease. It does this by lowering cholesterol, improving blood and oxygen supply to the heart, increasing the functional capacity of the heart, reducing blood pressure, reducing obesity, and exerting a favorable effect on blood clotting.[1]

Regular exercise makes people not only look better, but also makes them feel better. Tensions, depressions, feelings of inadequacy, and worries diminish greatly with regular exercise. The value of an exercise program in the treatment of depression cannot be overstated. Exercise alone has proved to have a tremendous impact on improving mood and the ability to handle stressful situations.

Exercise is so important to so many aspects of health that a summary of its benefits is in order.

Health Benefits of Exercise

Improved cardiovascular function: decreased heart rate, improved heart contraction, reduced blood pressure, and decreased blood cholesterol

Reduced secretions of adrenaline and noradrenaline, in response to psychological stress

Improved oxygen and nutrient utilization in all tissues

Increased self-esteem and improved mood and frame of mind

Increased endurance and energy

Relating Exercise and Sexual Performance   OK, so exercise is important, but will regular exercise improve a man's sexual performance? The answer to this question is yes. This answer is not just based on common sense, but also on clinical research. For example, one study researched the effects of nine months of regular exercise on aerobic work capacity (physical fitness), coronary heart disease risk factors, and sexuality. This study involved 78 sedentary but healthy men (mean age, 48 years).[14] The men exercised in supervised groups 60 minutes per day, 3.5 days per week, on average. Peak sustained exercise intensity was 75% to 80% of maximum heart rate. (The topic of maximum heart rate will be discussed later in this chapter.) A control group of 17 men (mean age, 44 years) participated in organized walking at a moderate pace for 60 minutes per day, 4.1 days per week, on average. During the first and last months of the program, each subject maintained a daily diary of exercise, diet, smoking, and sexuality. As in many other studies, the beneficial effects of regular exercise included increased fitness and a reduction in heart disease risk factors. Analysis of diary entries revealed significantly greater sexual benefits for exercisers than for nonexercisers. The benefits included increases in the frequency of various intimate activities, reliability of adequate functioning during sex, percentage of satisfying orgasms, and the like. Moreover, the degree of sexual benefit among exercisers was correlated with the degree of their individual improvement in fitness. In other words, the better physical fitness the men were able to attain, the better their sexuality.

Starting an Exercise Program   The first thing to do to start an exercise program is to make sure you are fit enough. If you have been mostly inactive for a number of years or have a previously diagnosed illness, see your physician first.

   If you are fit enough to begin, the next thing to do is select an activity that you feel you would enjoy. The best exercises are the kind that get your heart moving. Aerobic activities such as walking briskly, jogging, bicycling, cross-country skiing, swimming, aerobic dance, and racquet sports are examples. When you begin your program, brisk walking (5 miles an hour) for approximately 30 minutes may be the very best form of exercise.

Exercise intensity is determined by measuring your heart rate (the number of times your heart beats per minute). This can be quickly done by placing your index and middle fingers of one hand on the side of the neck just below the angle of the jaw or on the opposite wrist. Beginning with zero, count the number of heartbeats for 6 seconds. Simply add a zero to this number and you have your pulse rate per minute. For example, if you count 14 beats, your heart rate is 140 beats per minute. Is this a good number? It depends upon your training zone—the level of exercise that allows you to burn fat, without overworking.

A quick and easy way to determine your maximum training heart rate is simply to subtract your age from 185. For example, if you are 40 years old, your maximum heart rate is 145. To determine the bottom of the training zone, simply subtract 20 from your maximum heart rate. In the case of a 40-year-old, this is 125. So, exercise in the training zone produces a heart rate between 125 and 145 beats per minute. For maximum health benefits, you must stay in this range and never exceed it.

A minimum of 15 to 20 minutes of exercise, in your training zone and at least three times a week, is necessary to gain any significant benefit from exercise. It is better to exercise at the lower end of your training zone for longer periods of time than it is to exercise at a higher intensity for a shorter period of time.

The key to getting the maximum benefit from exercise is to make it fun. Choose an activity that you enjoy. If you can find enjoyment in exercise, you are much more likely to exercise regularly than someone who exercises from a sense of duty. You don't get in good physical condition by exercising once; exercise must be consistent. So, make it fun. Sex itself can be a form of exercise.

Plant-Based Medicines

In addition to nutritional measures and exercise, plant-based, or herbal, medicines are often used in the natural treatment of erectile dysfunction. Improving sexual desire and function is possible using plant-based medicines that (1) improve the activity of the male glandular system, (2) improve the blood supply to erectile tissue, and (3) enhance the transmission or stimulation of the nerve signal. Descriptions of several medicines that produce one or more of these effects follow in this chapter. Please read each description carefully. *The fact that a plant-based medicine is discussed here does not mean it is recommended for general use.* Also see Chapter 3, which discusses plant-based medicines in regard to infertility, and Chapter 8, which discusses the effects of *Panax ginseng.*

Using Yohimbe Bark   This chapter has already mentioned that the yohimbe tree (*Pausinystalia johimbe*) is the source of yohimbine, the only FDA-approved drug for the treatment of erectile dysfunction. Because of the yohimbine content of yohimbe bark, the FDA classifies yohimbe as an unsafe herb.[15] I think there is some validity to this classification. I have used yohimbine in my practice and have found that, because of side effects, it is very difficult to work with. Some men are much more sensitive to yohimbine than others. Because it is so powerful, yohimbe can produce the same kind of side effects as yohimbine. In my opinion, yohimbe and yohimbine are best used under the supervision of a physician. In addition to the problem of side effects caused by commercial yohimbe preparations, I am suspicious of the quality of yohimbe products in health food stores. To my knowledge, no commercial source of yohimbe bark available in a health food store actually states the level of yohimbine per dosage. Without knowing the content of yohimbine, prescribing an effective, safe, and consistent dosage is virtually impossible.

Using Muira Puama Extract   One of the best plants to use for erectile dysfunction or lack of libido is muira puama (*Ptychopetalum olacoides*), which is also known as potency wood. This shrub is native to Brazil and has long been used as a powerful aphrodisiac and nerve stimulant in South American folk medicine.[15] A recent clinical study has validated its safety and effectiveness in improving libido and sexual function in some patients.[16]

At the Institute of Sexology in Paris, France, Dr. Jacques Waynberg (one of the world's foremost authorities on sexual function) supervised a clinical study involving an extract of muira puama. The study involved 262 patients who complained of lack of sexual desire and the inability to attain or maintain an erection. Extract of muira puama was effective in helping many of these men. Within two weeks, at a daily dose of 1 to 1.5 grams of the extract, 62% of patients with loss of libido claimed that the treatment had dynamic effect; 51% of patients with "erection failures" felt that muira puama was of benefit.

Presently, no one knows for sure how muira puama improves sexual function. It seems to enhance both psychological and physical aspects. Future research will undoubtedly shed light on how the chemicals in this extremely helpful plant affect erectile dysfunction.

Using *Ginkgo biloba* Extract   Extract of *Ginkgo biloba*, a tree, is one of the most popular medicines in France and Germany. In Germany, over 5 million prescriptions are written each year for ginkgo extract. Most American physicians have never heard of it, and this is unfortunate because so many people in the United States could benefit from ginkgo extract. In the United States, ginkgo extract is available in health food stores.

Numerous clinical studies have demonstrated that ginkgo extract is extremely beneficial in treating vascular insufficiency. In clinical trials, patients with chronic cerebral arterial insufficiency and patients with peripheral arterial insufficiency have responded favorably to ginkgo extract.[17] Most of the time *Ginkgo biloba* extract is used to help elderly people whose blood flow to the brain is impaired. (This condition is known as cerebral insufficiency.) The symptoms of cerebral insufficiency include short-term memory loss, vertigo, headache, ringing in the ears, depression, and impotence (in males). These symptoms are often referred to as symptoms of aging.

A recent analysis reviewed the quality of the research in over 40 clinical studies that examined the effect of a standardized extract of *Ginkgo biloba* leaves on cerebral insufficiency.[18] The analysis indicated that the quality of the research was on a par with the research used in investigating the drug Hydergine (ergoloid mesylates). Hydergine is an FDA-approved drug for the treatment of dementia, including Alzheimer's disease. The analysis substantiated that ginkgo is effective in reducing all symptoms of cerebral insufficiency, including impaired mental function (senility). *Ginkgo biloba* extract has been extensively studied and appears to work by increasing blood flow to the brain, resulting in an increase in oxygen and glucose utilization.

In addition to its use in increasing blood and oxygen flow to the brain, recent evidence indicates that *Ginkgo biloba* extract may be extremely beneficial in the treatment of erectile dysfunction due to lack of blood flow.[19] One study involved 60 patients with proven erectile dysfunction who had not reacted to papaverine injections of up to 50 milligrams. These patients were treated with *Ginkgo biloba* extract in a dose of 60 milligrams per day, for 12 to 18 months. Penile blood flow was re-evaluated by duplex sonography every four weeks.

The first signs of improved blood supply were seen after six to eight weeks; after six months of therapy, 50% of the patients had regained potency. In 20%, a new trial of papaverine injection was then successful. In 25%, blood flow had improved but papaverine was still not successful. The blood flow of the remaining 5% was unchanged.

The improvement of the arterial inflow to erectile tissue is assumed to be due to the ability of *Ginkgo biloba* extract to enhance blood flow through arteries and veins, without changing systemic blood pressure.

Ginkgo's effects are more apparent with long-term therapy than short-term therapy, and some of the best results have been obtained by administering a dosage of 120 milligrams per day. The standard dosage of *Ginkgo biloba* extract is 40 milligrams, three times per day. To be sure the product you buy is of the same quality as that used in the clinical studies, make sure it contains 24% ginkgo heterosides (flavonglycosides). You can determine the concentration by reading the product label.

Using Damiana   The leaves of the damiana (*Turnera diffusa*) have been used in the United States since 1874 as an aphrodisiac and "to improve the sexual ability of the enfeebled and aged."[20] Although no clinical studies support this claim, damiana use is very popular. Damiana is thought to slightly irritate the urethra, thereby increasing the sensitivity of the penis.[20] Damiana is seldom used alone; most often it is recommended along with other commercial herbal preparations. If an individual desires the benefit of damiana on its own, drinking a daily cup of damiana tea should be sufficient to produce urethral irritation.

Chapter Summary

It is normal for a man to retain sexual function well into his 80s. However, erectile dysfunction is an extremely common condition that affects over 10 million American men. Restoring potency requires addressing the underlying cause. In the majority of cases, the cause is an organic factor. The chief cause is vascular insufficiency due to atherosclerosis.

There are a variety of medical treatments for erectile dysfunction, but each treatment has its drawbacks. The natural approach to erectile dysfunction involves the use of diet, exercise, nutritional supplements, and plant-based medicines. This approach is designed to restore potency by restoring normal physiology.

3

Male Infertility

E stimates state that as many as 15% of all couples in the United States have difficulty in conceiving a child. In about one-third of the cases of infertility, it is the man who is responsible; in another one-third, both male and female are responsible; and in another one-third, it is the female who is responsible. About 6% of men between the ages of 15 and 50 are infertile.[1]

Most cases of male infertility are the result of abnormal sperm count or quality. Although it takes only one sperm to fertilize an egg, an average ejaculate contains nearly 200 million sperm. The natural barriers in the female reproductive tract prevent all but about 40 sperm from reaching the vicinity of an egg. The number of sperm in an ejaculate and the degree of fertility are strongly correlated.

Deficient sperm production is the cause of about 90% of cases involving low sperm count. Unfortunately, in about 90% of these cases, the cause of deficient production cannot be identified and the condition is labeled idiopathic.[2] *Idiopathic* means resulting from an unknown cause.

Two conditions are associated with insufficient sperm: oligospermia and azoospermia. *Oligospermia* refers to a low sperm count; *azoospermia* refers to the complete absence of living sperm in the semen. Other causes of male infertility include ductal obstruction, ejaculatory dysfunction, infections, and disorders of accessory glands.

Since the overwhelming majority of men that are infertile suffer from deficient sperm production, this chapter will focus on that topic. If you are interested in other specific causes of infertility (see Figure 3.1), check the index of this book; other chapters discuss several other causes.

Sperm count as well as sperm quality has been deteriorating over the last few decades. In 1940, the average sperm count was 113 million per milliliter; by 1990, that value had dropped to 66 million.[3] Adding to this problem, the amount of semen fell almost 20%, from 3.4 milliliters

---

Deficient sperm production

Ductal obstruction
  Congenital defects
  Postinfectious obstruction
  Cystic fibrosis
  Vasectomy

Ejaculatory dysfunction
  Premature ejaculation
  Retrograde ejaculation

Disorders of accessory glands
  Infection
  Inflammation
  Antisperm antibodies

Coital disorders
  Defects in technique
  Premature withdrawal
  Erectile dysfunction

Figure 3.1   Causes of male infertility

Increased scrotal temperature
  Tight-fitting clothing and briefs
  Increase in varicoceles*

Increased pollution of the environment
  Heavy metals (lead, mercury, arsenic, etc.)
  Organic solvents
  Pesticides (DDT, PCBs, etc.)

Dietary degradation
  Increased intake of saturated fats
  Reduced intake of fruits, vegetables. and whole grains
  Reduced intake of dietary fiber
  Increased exposure to synthetic estrogen

*Varicose swellings that, when viewed through the skin of the scrotum, look blue.

Figure 3.2   Possible reasons sperm counts are falling

to 2.75 milliliters. Altogether these changes mean that, per ejaculate, men are now supplying only about 40% of the number of sperm men supplied in 1940.

The downward trend in sperm count has led to speculation that recent environmental, dietary, or lifestyle changes are interfering with a man's ability to manufacture sperm (see Figure 3.2). Although the speculation is controversial, substantial evidence supports it. This evidence and methods for improving sperm quality will be discussed later in this chapter.

Diagnosis of Male Infertility

Semen analysis is the test most widely used to estimate the fertility potential of a male. Keep in mind the fact that a low sperm count does not necessarily mean infertility, permanent or temporary. As Figure 3.3 shows, many factors can contribute to low counts that are temporary. When the cause disappears, so does the low count.

A semen analysis involves determining sperm concentration and sperm quality. During the last 40 years scientists have changed their minds about the concentration that differentiates infertile and fertile men. In 1950, the sperm concentration thought to define fertility was 40 million sperm per milliliter. Now it is 5 million per milliliter. The reason the definition has changed so drastically is that researchers are learning that sperm quality is more important than quantity. A high sperm count means absolutely nothing if the percentage of healthy sperm is not also high.

Whenever the majority of sperm are abnormally shaped or are entirely or relatively nonmotile, a man can be infertile despite having a normal sperm concentration. (Figure 3.4 shows the normal shape and typical abnormal shapes for sperm.) Conversely, a low sperm count does not always mean a man is infertile. Numerous men having very low sperm counts are now biological fathers. For example, in studies at fertility clinics, 52% of couples whose sperm counts were below 10 million per milliliter achieved pregnancy; 40% of those with sperm counts as low as 5 million per milliliter achieved pregnancy.[1] The success of these men with low sperm counts conveys a significant

---

High scrotal temperature

Infections (the common cold, the flu, etc.)

Severe stress

Lack of sleep

Overuse of alcohol, tobacco, or marijuana

Many prescription drugs

Exposure to radiation

Exposure to solvents, pesticides, and other toxins

Figure 3.3   Causes of temporary low sperm count

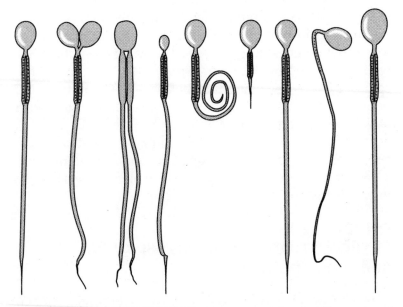

Figure 3.4 Abnormal infertile sperm compared with a normal sperm, on the right

lesson: Interpret the results of conventional semen analysis with caution in regard to the likelihood of conception. Use tests that are more sophisticated than semen analysis, especially when being screened (as part of a couple) for in vitro fertilization. The next two paragraphs will discuss these tests.

Until relatively recently, pregnancy was the only proof of the ability of sperm to achieve fertilization. Now a post-coital test can measure the ability of sperm to penetrate the cervical mucus. Test-tube variants of this test are available. Another type of test is based on the discovery that human sperm, under appropriate conditions, can penetrate hamster eggs. From 10% to 100% of sperm from a fertile human male can penetrate hamster eggs. If less than 10% of the sperm penetrate, infertility is indicated.

Hamster egg penetration can predict fertility in 66% of cases; semen analysis can predict fertility in only 30% of cases.[1]

Another important test in the diagnosis of infertility is a test that detects antisperm antibodies. These antibodies, when produced by the man, usually attack the tail of the sperm, thereby impeding the sperm's ability to move and penetrate the cervical mucus. In contrast, the antisperm antibodies produced by a woman are typically directed against the head. The presence of antisperm antibodies in semen analysis is usually a sign of past or current infection in the male reproductive tract. (The role of infections in male infertility will be discussed in Chapter 5.)

Medical Treatment of Oligospermia and Azoospermia

Medical treatment of low sperm count, or oligospermia, can be quite effective when the cause is known. Examples of causes are high scrotal temperature, chronic infection of male sex glands, prescription medicines, and endocrine disturbances. Treatment is directed at the underlying cause. However, as you have learned, in about 90% of the cases of oligospermia, the cause is unknown; the condition is called idiopathic oligospermia.

In regard to the absence of living sperm in the semen, or azoospermia, one cause may be ductal obstruction. If this is the case, new surgical techniques are producing positive results.[1]

The Importance of Scrotal Temperature

The scrotal sac is supposed to keep the testes at a temperature between 94 and 96 degrees Fahrenheit.[2] If the temperature rises above 96 degrees, sperm production is greatly inhibited or stopped completely. Typically, the mean scrotal temperature of infertile men is significantly higher than that of fertile men. Reducing the scrotal temperature of infertile men is often enough to make them fertile. The man may be able to reduce his scrotal temperature simply by not wearing tight-fitting underwear or jeans and avoiding hot tubs.

Some exercises can raise scrotal temperature—especially if, when he does them, a man is wearing synthetic fabrics, tight shorts, or tight bikini underwear. These exercises include rowing in a rowing machine, simulated cross-country skiing, using a treadmill, and jogging. In addition to avoiding clothing that can raise scrotal temperature, a man should allow his testicles to hang free after exercising. This allows them to recover from heat buildup.

Infertile men should wear boxer-type underwear. If they are serious about wanting to conceive, they should periodically apply ice or take cold showers to apply cold water to the scrotum. They can also use a device called a testicular hypothermia device, or "testicle cooler," to reduce scrotal temperature. Still in a somewhat primitive stage, the testicle cooler looks like a jockstrap from which long, thin tubes extend. The tubes are attached to a small fluid reservoir filled with cold water. The reservoir attaches to a belt around the waist. A pump in the reservoir causes the water to circulate. When the water reaches the surface of the scrotum, it evaporates and keeps the scrotum cool. Because of evaporation, the reservoir must be filled every six hours or so. It is recommended that the testicle cooler be worn daily, during waking hours. Most users claim that it is fairly comfortable and easy to conceal.[4]

Increased scrotal temperature can be due to the presence of a varicocele (a swelling caused by varicose veins in the scrotum). A large varicocele can cause the scrotum to reach too high a temperature for sperm production or motility. Surgical repair may be necessary, but be sure to try the program this section has described before electing to have surgery. And, make sure you get a second opinion to make sure that the varicocele is severe enough to be responsible for the elevated temperature.

The Natural Approach to Oligospermia and Azoospermia

Like the standard medical approach, the natural approach to oligospermia and azoospermia addresses the underlying causes. If high scrotal temperature is responsible, follow the recommendations cited in the previous section. If there is an infection, follow the recommendations in Chapter 5. If there is a blockage in sperm transport, it will have to be cleared. If a man is hypothyroid or not producing enough testosterone, follow the recommendations later in this chapter, in the section called "Means for Countering Estrogens."

In the treatment of so-called idiopathic oligospermia or azoospermia, the natural approach focuses on enhancing factors that promote sperm formation. In addition to scrotal temperature, sperm formation is closely linked to nutrition. This fact is undeniable. Therefore, it is critical that men with low sperm counts have optimal nutritional intake. The diet and nutritional supplement program discussed in Chapters 6 and 7 provides a strong nutritional foundation. Several nutritional factors deserve special mention in this chapter: vitamin C and other antioxidants, zinc, vitamin B12, arginine, and carnitine. You will read more about them in the sections that follow. In addition, you will read about the negative effects of estrogens and certain fats and oils and how to avoid or counter them.

Plant-Based Medicines

The natural approach to oligospermia and azoospermia includes the use of plant-based, or herbal, medicines. The best choice, from the standpoints of effect and availability, is a high-quality standardized product derived from *Panax ginseng*. Chapter 8 will discuss the effects of this plant in detail. Besides *Panax ginseng*, a number of Chinese herbal formulas have produced impressive clinical results. Most notable are Hachimijiogan, Ninjintoh, Hochu-Ekki-To, and Goshajinkigan. These mixtures are not readily available in the United States. They may be available at some Chinese herb shops or through an acupuncturist, however. Another Chinese plant that may be useful is *Astragalus membraneceus*. Because of its impressive immunity-enhancing effects, astragalus is now widely available in U.S. health food stores. Astragalus has been shown to enhance sperm motility in test-tube experiments and may have a similar effect in the body.[5] A dosage of 500 milligrams of astragalus, three times per day, may be useful in cases of reduced sperm motility—especially if the reduction is due to an infection.

Glandular Therapy

Another popular natural treatment for male infertility involves the use of glandular therapy. For almost as long as records have been kept, glandular therapy has been an important form of medicine. The basic concept underlying the medicinal use of glandular substances from animals is that like heals like. For example, if your liver needs support or you are suffering from liver disease, then you may benefit from eating beef liver. To correct low testosterone or a low sperm count, extracts of the orchic, or testicular, tissues of bulls are often recommended. It is well established that a number of glandular preparations are effective orally because they contain active hormones. Dosage as well as effectiveness varies from one preparation to another. Use well-respected brands and follow the dosage recommendations given by the manufacturer.

Means for Countering Estrogens

According to experts on the impact of the environment and diet on fetal development, we now live in an environment that can be viewed as "a virtual sea of estrogens."[6,7] (The plural, "estrogens," is used here because the body produces several types of estrogen. What is more, the estrogen substances found in the environment are not all from human sources. Some are from animals; others are synthetic and are found in pesticides and birth control pills, for example.) Increased exposure to estrogens during fetal development as well as during reproductive years may be a major cause of the tremendous increase in the developmental disorders and malfunctions of the male sexual system.

The relationship between estrogens and male sexual development is best viewed by discussing a synthetic estrogen, diethylstilbesterol (DES). DES is now recognized to have led to substantial increases in developmental problems of the reproductive tract as well as low semen volume and sperm count.[6] As well as being used in humans, DES and other synthetic estrogens were used for about 30 years in the livestock industry, to fatten animals and help them grow faster.

Although many synthetic estrogens are now outlawed, as DES is, livestock and poultry are still hormonally manipulated, especially dairy cows. Because of modern farming techniques, cow's milk contains substantial amounts of estrogen. The rise in dairy consumption since the 1940s inversely parallels the drop in human sperm production. Avoidance of hormone-fed animal products and milk products is an absolute must for male sexual vitality—especially for men with low sperm counts or testosterone levels.

There are reports that estrogens have been detected in drinking water.[6,7] Presumably, the estrogens are recycled, at water treatment plants, from excreted synthetic estrogens (such as birth control pills). These estrogens may be extremely harmful to male sexual vitality, because they are more potent than natural human estrogen. Their potency results from the fact that they do not bind to sex-hormone–binding globulin (SHBG). Drinking purified or bottled water may be a suitable way to prevent exposure to estrogen in the public water supply.

Other sources of estrogen in the environment (food, water, and air) can weaken male sexual vitality. For example, many of the chemicals with which we have contaminated our environment in the past 50 years are weakly estrogenic. Most of these chemicals—such as PCBs, dioxin, and DDT— are resistant to biodegradation and are recycled in the environment until they find safe haven in our bodies. For example, even though DDT has been banned for nearly 20 years, it is still often found in the soil and in root vegetables such as carrots and potatoes. (For more on this subject, see *The Healing Power of Foods,* by Michael T. Murray, Prima Publishing, Rocklin, California, 1993.) Many toxic chemicals are known to interfere with spermato-genesis, but their effects on sexual development may be even more significant.

All the estrogenic sources discussed so far are thought to have their greatest impact during fetal development. Animal studies show that estrogens inhibit the multiplication of the Sertoli cells. Remember, these cells support, protect, and regulate the nutrition of the developing sperm. The number of Sertoli cells is directly proportional to the amount of sperm that can be produced. Each Sertoli cell can only support a fixed number of germ cells that will develop into sperm. Therefore, the lower the number of Sertoli cells, the lower the number of sperm that can be produced.

Sertoli cell multiplication occurs primarily during fetal life and before puberty. It is controlled by follicle-stimulating hormone (FSH). In animal studies, estrogens administered early in life inhibit FSH secretion, resulting in a low number of Sertoli cells and, in adult life, a low sperm count. Evidence indicates that the same events occur in humans.[6] The sons of women exposed to DES during pregnancy provide an example of the results of the process in humans. Like the animals exposed to estrogens, these men have low sperm counts.

If you are an adult male, there isn't a lot that can be done about the environment that you were exposed to while in your mother's womb. Even if your mother didn't take DES, she may have followed the typical low-fiber, high-fat diet of most Americans. Such a diet is associated with high levels of estrogens—without the fiber, excreted estrogens are simply reabsorbed. Regardless of the reason you may not be producing enough sperm, however, dietary practices can ensure that your sperm-producing capabilities are at their maximum. Just follow the recommendations in this chapter and in Chapters 6 and 7.

In particular, if your testosterone level is low or marginal or if your estrogen level is elevated, eat a diet rich in legumes (beans)—especially soy foods. Soy is a particularly good source of isoflavonoids. These compounds are also known as phytoestrogens, a name that indicates their mild estrogenic activity. The isoflavonoids in soybeans have about 0.2% of the estrogen activity of estradiol, the principal human estrogen. Isoflavonoids actually bind to estrogen receptors. Their weak estrogenic action is in actuality an anti-estrogenic effect, because it prevents the body's own estrogen from binding to the receptor. In addition, phytoestrogens may reduce the effects of estrogens by stimulating the production of SHBG so that the estrogen is bound.[8] Soy—as well as legumes, nuts, and seeds—is also a good source of phytosterols. The significance of this is explained in Chapter 6.

Vitamin C and Other Antioxidants

The cells of the human body are constantly under attack. The culprits: free radicals and pro-oxidants. These highly reactive molecules can bind to and destroy cellular components. A free radical is a molecule that contains a highly reactive unpaired electron; a pro-oxidant is a molecule that can promote oxidative damage. Free radical or oxidative damage is what makes us age. Free radicals have also been shown to be responsible for many diseases—including the two biggest killers of Americans, heart disease and cancer. And, free radical damage to sperm is thought to be responsible for many cases of so-called idiopathic oligospermia.[9]

Where do these sinister free radicals come from? Believe it or not, most of the free radicals zipping through our bodies are actually produced during normal metabolic processes—energy production, detoxification reactions, and immune defense. The environment contributes to an individual's free radical load. Cigarette smoking increases it further. Other external sources of free radicals include ionizing radiation, chemotherapeutic drugs, air pollutants, pesticides, anesthetics, aromatic hydrocarbons, solvents, alcohol, and formaldehyde.

Men exposed to these sources of free radicals are much more likely to have abnormal sperm and sperm counts than men who are not exposed.[1, 9-12] High levels of free radicals are found in the semen of 40% of infertile men.[13] Sperm are particularly susceptible to free radical damage, as well as the damaging effects of heavy metals such as lead, cadmium, arsenic, and mercury. All men with reduced sperm counts should undergo a hair mineral analysis for heavy metals. The analysis will determine if heavy metals are contributing to or causing the problem.

Cigarette smoking is closely associated with low sperm counts, poor sperm motility, and a high frequency of abnormal sperm.[12] Cigarette smoking, as well as the increase in environmental pollution, are thought to be major contributors to the decrease in human sperm production in many industrialized nations during the past few decades.

Sperm are extremely sensitive to free radicals because sperm are so dependent upon the integrity and fluidity of the cell membrane. Low fluidity activates enzymes and events that can lead to impaired motility; abnormal structure; loss of viability; and, ultimately, the death of the sperm.[9]

The major determinant of membrane fluidity is the presence of polyunsaturated fatty acids—particularly, omega-3 fatty acids, such as docosahexanoic acid. Unfortunately, unsaturated acids are very susceptible to free radical damage. The sperm do not have the luxury that many other cells throughout the body have; sperm have a relative lack of the enzymes that prevent or repair oxidative damage. Adding to this compromised state is the fact that sperm generate high quantities of free radicals to help break down barriers to fertilization. To summarize, three factors render sperm particularly susceptible to free radical damage: (1) a high concentration of polyunsaturated fatty acids, (2) a lack of defensive enzymes, and (3) active generation of free radicals. These factors make the health of the sperm critically dependent upon antioxidants.

Antioxidants are compounds that help protect against free radical damage. Antioxidants—such as vitamin C, beta-carotene, selenium, and vitamin E—protect against the development of heart disease and cancer and are thought to slow the aging process. These nutrients also play critical roles in sperm formation.

Vitamin C (ascorbic acid), perhaps the most well studied antioxidant, plays an especially important role in protecting the sperm's genetic material (DNA) from damage. The ascorbic acid level in seminal fluid is much higher than that in other body fluids, including the blood. In one study involving healthy human subjects, dietary vitamin C was reduced from 250 milligrams to 5 milligrams per day. As a result, the ascorbic acid in seminal fluid decreased by 50% and the number of sperm with damaged DNA increased by 91%.[14] These results underline the facts that dietary vitamin C plays a critical role in protecting against sperm damage and that a low level of dietary vitamin C is likely to lead to infertility.

It is now a well-known fact that cigarette smoking greatly reduces vitamin C throughout the body. The Food and Nutrition Board, the organization that calculates the Recommended Dietary Allowances (RDAs), acknowledges that smokers require at least twice as much vitamin C as nonsmokers.[15] One of the reasons a smoker may have a reduced sperm count is vitamin C depletion. In one study, men who smoked one pack of cigarettes a day received either 0, 200, or 1,000 milligrams of vitamin C. After one month, sperm quality improved in proportion to the level of vitamin C supplementation—that is to say, as the level of vitamin C increased, so did sperm quality.[16]

Nonsmokers appear to benefit as much from vitamin C as smokers. In one study, 30 infertile but otherwise healthy men received either 200 milligrams or 1,000 milligrams of vitamin C or placebo daily.[17] Weekly measurements established sperm count, viability, motility, agglutination, abnormalities, and immaturity. After one week, the 1,000-milligram group demonstrated a 140% increase in sperm count; the 200-milligram group, a 112% increase; and the placebo group, no change. After three weeks, both vitamin C groups continued to improve; the improvement of the 200-milligram group caught up to that of the 1,000-milligram group. One of the key improvements involved the number of agglutinated sperm. Sperm become agglutinated when antibodies produced by the immune system bind to it. Antibodies to sperm are often associated with chronic genito-urinary tract or prostatic infection. When more than 25% of the sperm are agglutinated, fertility is very unlikely. At the beginning of the study, all three groups had over 25% agglutinated sperm. After three weeks, only 11% of the sperm in the vitamin C groups were agglutinated. Although this result is impressive, the most impressive result of the study was that, at the end of 60 days, all men in the vitamin C group had impregnated their wives. None of the men in the placebo group had done so. These results clearly show that vitamin C supplementation can be very effective in treating male infertility, especially if the infertility is due to antibodies against sperm.

Other dietary antioxidants—such as vitamin E, selenium, and beta-carotene—are also important. Supplement your intake according to the guidelines in Chapter 7. Vitamin E supplementation appears especially warranted because it is the main antioxidant in various cell membranes, including sperm membranes. Vitamin E also plays an essential role in inhibiting free radical damage to the unsaturated fatty acids of the sperm membrane.[18] In addition, vitamin E enhances the ability of sperm to fertilize an egg in test tubes. Vitamin E supplementation at a dosage of 300 international units (IUs) per day has not been shown to improve sperm counts or motility.[19] However, supplementation appears to be indicated based on its physiological effects alone. My recommendation for infertile men is 600 to 800 international units of vitamin E per day. Vitamin E, in this amount, may prove to exert beneficial effects on sperm count and motility.

In addition to nutritional supplements of antioxidants, a diet high in fruits, vegetables, and legumes is critical. These foods are rich sources of components that cause potent antioxidant activity. Follow the dietary recommendations given in Chapter 6 to ensure a high intake of antioxidants.

Reduced Saturate Intake, Increased Polyunsaturate Intake

Infertile men should avoid certain fats but increase their intake of others. In short, saturated fats should be avoided. These fats are found primarily in animal products, especially butter and lard. Do not use margarine; shortening; or coconut, palm, or cottonseed oil. Coconut and palm oils are primarily saturated fat. Cottonseed oil may contain toxic residues, because cotton is so heavily sprayed. In addition, cottonseed oil is a rich source of gossypol, a substance known to inhibit sperm function. In fact, gossypol is being investigated as the "male birth control pill." Its use as an antifertility agent began after studies demonstrated that men who had used crude cottonseed oil as cooking oil had low sperm counts followed by total testicular failure.[20] Read food labels carefully to avoid all sources of cottonseed oil.

While the intake of saturated and hydrogenated fats must be eliminated, the intake of polyunsaturated oils should be increased. These oils function in all aspects of sexual function, including sperm formation and activity. Perhaps the best way to increase the intake of these vital oils is by the regular consumption of nuts and seeds (see Chapter 6). When consumption of polyunsaturated fats increases, so does the need for vitamin E. The relationship between polyunsaturated fats and vitamin E provides good reason to supplement your diet with vitamin E.

Zinc

Zinc is perhaps the most critical trace mineral for male sexual function. It is involved in virtually every aspect of male reproduction, including hormone metabolism, sperm formation, and sperm motility.[21] Zinc deficiency is characterized by, among many other things, decreased testosterone levels and sperm counts. Zinc levels are typically much lower in infertile men with low sperm counts than in fertile men with normal sperm counts. This indicates that a low zinc status may be the contributing factor to the infertility.

Several studies have measured the effect of zinc supplementation on sperm counts and motility.[22-24] The results from all the studies support the use of zinc supplementation in the treatment of oligospermia, especially when the testosterone level is low. The effectiveness of zinc is best illustrated by the results of a study that involved 37 men with infertility of greater than 5 years' duration and whose sperm counts were less than 25 million per milliliter. Blood testosterone levels were also measured.[24] The men received a supplement of zinc sulfate (60 milligrams of elemental zinc daily) for 45 to 50 days. In the 22 patients with initially low testosterone levels, mean sperm count increased significantly. The increase ranged from 8 to 20 million. Testosterone levels also increased, and 9 out of 22 wives became pregnant during the study. This result is quite impressive given the long-term nature of the infertility and the immediate results. In contrast, in the 15 men with normal testosterone levels, sperm count increased slightly, but there was no change in testosterone level and no pregnancies occurred.

Optimal zinc levels must be attained if optimum male sexual vitality is desired. Although severe zinc deficiency is quite rare in the United States, many men consume a diet that is low in zinc. The RDA is 15 milligrams for men and 12 milligrams for women. Zinc is found in significant amounts in whole grains, legumes, nuts, and seeds. In addition to eating these zinc-containing foods, take a daily multiple vitamin that contains sufficient zinc (see Chapter 7).

Vitamin B12

Vitamin B12 is involved in cellular replication. A deficiency of B12 leads to reduced sperm count and sperm motility. Even in the absence of a vitamin B12 deficiency, supplementation appears to be worthwhile for men with sperm counts of less than 20 million per milliliter or a motility rate of less than 50%. In one study, men with sperm counts of less than 20 million took 1,000 micrograms per day of vitamin B12. Of these men, 27% were able to achieve a total count in excess of 100 million.[25] In another study, men with low sperm counts took 6,000 micrograms per day. Of these men, 57% showed improvements.[26]

Arginine

The amino acid arginine is required for the replication of cells, making it essential in sperm formation. Arginine supplementation is often, but not always, an effective treatment of male infertility. The critical determinate appears to be the degree of oligospermia. If the sperm count is less than 20 million per milliliter, arginine supplementation is less likely to be of benefit than in cases where the count is higher. To be effective, it appears that the dosage of L-arginine be at least 4 grams a day, for three months. (Note that the dosage cites L-arginine, a specific form.) In perhaps the most favorable study, L-arginine caused significant improvement in 74% of 178 men with low sperm counts; sperm counts and motility increased.[27] Because arginine therapy is expensive, do not use it until after other nutritional measures have been tried.

Carnitine

Carnitine is a vitaminlike compound that stimulates mitochondria (the cell components that produce energy) to break down long-chain fatty acids. Carnitine is essential in the transport of fatty acids into the mitochondria. A deficiency in carnitine results in a decrease in fatty acid concentrations in the mitochondria and reduced energy production.

Carnitine concentrations are extremely high in the epididymis and sperm, suggesting that carnitine plays a role in male reproductive function. The epididymis derives the majority of its energy requirements from fatty acids. So do the sperm, as they travel through the epididymis. After ejaculation, the motility of sperm correlates positively with carnitine content. The higher the carnitine content, the more motile the sperm.[28]

Since carnitine can be synthesized from the essential amino acid lysine, many nutritionists and researchers have argued that it should not be considered a vitamin. Others argue that if niacin (which can be synthesized from the essential amino acid tryptophan) can be labeled a vitamin, then so should carnitine.

Carnitine can be helpful in fighting many diseases. The best clinical applications, however, involve cardiovascular diseases. Normal heart function is critically dependent on adequate concentrations of carnitine. Having a deficiency of carnitine in the heart is similar to trying to run an automobile without a fuel pump: There may be plenty of fuel, but there is no way to get it to the engine. The normal heart stores more carnitine than it needs. If the heart does not have a good supply of oxygen, carnitine levels quickly decrease. This lack of oxygen leads to decreased energy production in the heart and increased risk for angina and heart disease. Since angina patients have a decreased supply of oxygen, carnitine supplementation makes sense. Several clinical trials have demonstrated that carnitine improves angina and heart disease.[28] Supplementation with carnitine normalizes heart carnitine levels and allows the heart muscle to utilize its limited oxygen supply more efficiently.

Presumably, a similar scenario exists in some men with low sperm counts. A low carnitine level means that sperm development, function, and motility are drastically reduced. Supplementing the diet with L-carnitine may be useful in restoring male fertility. The optimal dosage is 300 to 1,000 milligrams, three times daily. It is important to use L-carnitine instead of D,L-carnitine, which is a mixture of the D and L forms of carnitine. The body uses L-carnitine; D-carnitine actually interferes with L-carnitine. Because L-carnitine is expensive, try other nutritional measures before investing in L-carnitine.

Chapter Summary

Male infertility is most often due to an insufficient number of sperm or poor semen quality. Exposure to estrogens during fetal development may explain the increase in the male reproductive abnormalities and reduced sperm counts seen during the last 50 years.

Sperm formation is closely linked to nutrition and antioxidant status. Since sperm are particularly susceptible to free radical and oxidative damage, avoid environmental sources of free radicals and eat a diet rich in antioxidants. Nutrients critical to healthy sperm include vitamin C and other antioxidants, essential fatty acids, zinc, vitamin B12, arginine, and L-carnitine.

Prostate Health

I mproving prostate health is a critical goal when trying to improve sexual function, including erectile dysfunction and male infertility. Proper prostate function is essential for normal reproductive function. Unfortunately, disorders of the prostate are extremely common in American men.

Enlargement of the prostate (benign prostatic hyperplasia, or BPH) affects more than half of all American men over 40 years of age; about 10% of American men will develop prostate cancer in their lifetime, and about one-quarter of these men will die from it. Inflammation or infection of the prostate (prostatitis) is also quite common.

Because an enlarged or cancerous prostate can pinch off the flow of urine, both BPH and prostate cancer are characterized by symptoms of bladder obstruction: increased urinary frequency, nighttime awakening to an empty bladder, and reduced force and caliber of urination. Prostatitis is associated with fever, penile discharge, and pain during urination.

Note: Prostate disorders can only be diagnosed by a physician. Do not self-diagnose. If you are experiencing any symptoms associated with BPH or prostate cancer, see your physician immediately for proper diagnosis.

Diagnosis of Prostate Disorders

Doctors often recommend that men over the age of 40 have a yearly digital prostate exam. This is not a high-tech test. A doctor simply inserts a gloved finger into the rectum and feels the lower part of the prostate for any abnormality. However, in the case of BPH, the prostate may not yet be enlarged to a point recognizable by digital exam. And, in the case of cancer, a digital exam is not reliable enough.

To a doctor performing a digital exam, the classic prostate enlarged because of BPH feels softer than normal (boggy) and may be two to three times larger than normal. BPH does not usually cause the prostate to feel tender to the patient. This differentiates it from prostatitis, which can be uncomfortable or painful. To the doctor performing an exam, a cancerous prostate feels much harder than usual and its border is not as well defined.

The definitive diagnosis for BPH can be made with ultrasound. For prostatitis, a urine sample or prostatic fluid examination often shows characteristic signs of infection or inflammation. For prostate cancer, a biopsy provides the definitive diagnosis.

In contrast to the classic cases, some cases of BPH and prostate cancer involve symptoms that are quite similar. A simple blood test is often used to differentiate the two. The blood test measures the levels of a protein that is produced in the prostate, prostate-specific antigen (PSA). The PSA test has been regarded as a highly significant and sensitive marker of prostate cancer. The normal value for PSA is less than 4 nanograms per milliliter. (A nanogram is one-billionth of a gram.) An elevation above 10 is highly indicative of prostate cancer.

There has been recent concern that the PSA test for prostate cancer is not reliable enough. Although an elevated PSA level does indicate prostate cancer in about 90% of cases, midrange elevations of PSA can be caused by BPH. In some instances, the prostate may be cancerous but PSA levels are not elevated. Despite the fact that the PSA test is not perfect, it is a simple, relatively noninvasive test that can provide valuable information. PSA screening has been endorsed by the American Cancer Society, the American Urological Association, and other physicians' groups.

If you are a man over the age of 50 and if any of your immediate relatives—father, brother, or uncle—has had prostate cancer, an annual prostate exam and PSA test is a very good idea.

Reduction of Prostate Cancer Risk

Several dietary factors have been shown to increase the likelihood of developing prostate cancer. The most significant causes are high intake of refined sugar, animal fat, and animal protein and a lack of carotenes.[1] A diet rich in plant foods and low in animal foods should offer some protection against prostatic cancer, especially if the intake of carotenes is high.[2]

Carotenes (also known as carotenoids) are a highly colored (red to yellow) group of fat-soluble compounds that protect plants against free radical damage produced during photosynthesis. Carotenes are best known for their capacity to convert into vitamin A, their antioxidant activity, and their anticancer properties. Low intake of carotene, specifically beta-carotene, is the most significant risk factor for prostate cancer.[2] The leading sources of carotenes are dark-green leafy vegetables (kale, collards, and spinach) and yellow-orange fruits and vegetables (apricots, cantaloupe, carrots, sweet potatoes, yams, and squash).

Following a high-fiber, vegetable-rich, and lowfat diet has been shown to enhance survivability in patients with metastatic prostate cancer (stage D2).[3] This finding is quite significant as part of a body of evidence that suggests that the best medical treatment in many cases of prostate cancer is no treatment.[4]

Medical Treatment of BPH and Prostatitis

If left untreated, BPH will eventually obstruct the bladder outlet, resulting in the retention of urine in the blood (uremia). Because uremia is a potentially life-threatening condition, proper treatment is crucial. In the past, medical treatment involved a procedure known as a TURP (trans-urethral resection of the prostate). This surgery is associated with complications and will often make matters worse, so it should be avoided unless absolutely necessary.

Finasteride (also known by the product name Proscar) is currently the only approved drug for the treatment of BPH. It works by inhibiting the activity of an enzyme, 5-alpha-reductase, involved in testosterone metabolism. Finasteride blocks the transformation of testosterone to dihydrotestosterone, a very potent hormone derived from testosterone. Dihydrotestosterone is responsible for the overproduction of prostate cells, which ultimately results in prostatic enlargement.

Proscar has received much attention. Based on the results of clinical trials, however, it is much less effective than an extract of *Serenoa repens* (discussed later in this chapter) and the other natural alternatives to be mentioned in the sections that follow. Less than 50% of patients on Proscar experience clinical improvement after taking the drug for one year; it must be taken for at least six months before any improvement can be expected. Proscar costs about $75 a month. Merck, the company that manufactures the drug, has predicted sales will soon reach $1 billion dollars annually.

In the case of prostatitis, the usual treatment is antibiotics. When treated with antibiotics alone, the condition is typically chronic and difficult to clear.

The Natural Approach to BPH and Prostatitis

Diet plays a critical role in the health of the prostate. Particularly important are zinc and essential fatty acids. A diet rich in zinc and essential fatty acids can improve and protect the prostate. Avoiding pesticides and keeping the cholesterol level below 200 milligrams per deciliter are also important. In many cases, these recommendations alone will bring about clinical improvement in BPH as well as chronic prostatitis. If additional support is necessary, several natural products can help. The fat-soluble extract of saw palmetto berries appears to be the best treatment for BPH; flower pollen extract is the natural treatment of choice for prostatitis. This section will discuss each of these components of the natural approach, plus a few more. For further suggestions about treating prostate infections, see Chapter 5.

Avoidance of Pesticides

In trying to treat or prevent BPH, as well as improve overall prostate health, the diet should be as free as possible from pesticides and other contaminants. Many of these compounds (such as dioxin, polyhalogenated biphenyls, hexachlorobenzene, and dibenzofurans) become concentrated within the prostate and can ultimately lead to BPH.[5] Any meat eaten should be free of synthetic hormones.

Synthetic hormones fed to animals to fatten them before slaughter have been shown to produce, in rat prostates, results similar to those of BPH.[5]

It is quite possible that the tremendous increase in BPH in the last few decades reflects an ever-increasing effect of toxic chemicals on our health. A diet rich in natural whole foods may offer some protection because whole foods contain many protective substances. These substances include, in particular, minerals (such as calcium, magnesium, zinc, and selenium), vitamins, plant pigments (flavonoids, carotenes, and chlorophyll, for example), fiber (especially gel-forming and mucilaginous types), and sulfur-containing compounds. All these can help the body deal with toxic chemicals and heavy metals.

Zinc and Essential Fatty Acids

Paramount to overall prostate health and effective BPH prevention and treatment is adequate zinc intake and absorption. In addition to being critical to testosterone synthesis and action and sperm formation, zinc is critical to prostate function. The prostate concentrates, then secretes, zinc. Zinc affects sperm motility and prevents infection. In fact, the prostate has the highest concentration of zinc of any body tissue. Frequent prostate infections may be a sign of a lack of zinc within the prostate.

In regard to BPH, rectal examination, x-ray films, and endoscopy show that zinc supplementation can reduce the size of the prostate.[6] In addition, research shows that zinc supplementation can reduce symptoms for the majority of BPH patients.[6] The clinical efficacy of zinc is probably due to its critical involvement in many aspects of hormonal metabolism.

Foods rich in zinc include nuts and seeds. These foods also provide an excellent source of essential fatty acids which, like zinc, are associated with positive results in the treatment of BPH. In one study, the administration of a mixture of essential fatty acids to 19 subjects with BPH showed a reduction in the amount of residual urine in the bladder.[7] In 12 of the 19, there was no residual urine by the end of several weeks of treatment. These effects appear to be due to the correction of an underlying essential fatty acid deficiency.[8] Based on this evidence alone, BPH patients should increase the intake of nuts and seeds or take zinc supplements and/or essential fatty acids.

A folk remedy for BPH is to eat ¼ to ½ cup of pumpkin seeds each day. Because pumpkin seeds are high in zinc and essential fatty acids, this appears to be a very sound recommendation. Vegetable oils that can healthfully meet the body's requirement for essential fatty acids include flaxseed oil, sunflower oil, evening primrose oil, and soy oil. Just 1 tablespoon per day is usually a sufficient amount.

Control of Cholesterol

Products resulting from the breakdown of cholesterol have been shown to accumulate in prostate tissue affected with either BPH or cancer.[5] These metabolites of cholesterol initiate degeneration of prostatic cells, which can promote prostatic enlargement. Drugs that lower cholesterol levels have been shown to have a favorable influence on BPH. The drugs prevent the accumulation of cholesterol in the prostatic cells and limit subsequent formation of damaging cholesterol metabolites. These facts suggest that, for prostate health, a man should make every effort to keep his total cholesterol level below 200 milligrams per deciliter.

Avoidance of Beer

Beer has been linked to BPH. Research suggests that beer increases the release of the hormone prolactin by the pituitary gland.[9] Prolactin increases the uptake of testosterone and its conversion, within the prostate, to dihydrotestosterone. Drugs that reduce prolactin, such as bromocryptine, reduce many of the symptoms of BPH. However, these drugs have severe side effects and are, therefore, not widely used. Fortunately, zinc and vitamin B6 can reduce prolactin and, at prescribed dosages, produce no side effects.[10,11]

Use of Saw Palmetto Berry Extract

Saw palmetto (*Serenoa repens*) is a small scrubby palm tree native to the West Indies and the Atlantic Coast of North America, from South Carolina to Florida. It bears berries that have a long folk history as an aphrodisiac and sexual rejuvenator. These berries have also been used for centuries in treating conditions of the prostate. This historical use led to the development of a purified fat-soluble extract that contains from 85% to 95% fatty acids and sterols. Over a dozen double-blind clinical studies have shown that this extract greatly improves symptoms of enlarged prostate.

Like Proscar, the therapeutic effect of the saw palmetto extract appears to be due to its inhibition of dihydrotestosterone, the compound that causes the prostate cells to multiply excessively. However, saw palmetto extract goes well beyond Proscar. The extract not only inhibits the formation of dihydrotestosterone, it also inhibits dihydrotestosterone from binding at cellular binding sites. Since Proscar has no effect on binding, saw palmetto has a much greater effect than Proscar—as clinical results prove.

Numerous studies show that saw palmetto extract is effective in nearly 90% of patients, usually in a period of four to six weeks.[12-21] In contrast, Proscar is effective in reducing the symptoms in less than 50% of patients who took it for one year. To illustrate saw palmetto extract's superiority over Proscar, look at the effect of both on the maximum urine flow rate (a good indicator of bladder neck

Table 4.1   Effects of Saw Palmetto Versus Effects of Proscar on Urine Flow Rate (ml/sec)

	Saw Palmetto Extract	Proscar
Initial measurement	9.53	9.60
3 months	13.15*	10.40
12 months	**	11.20
Percentage increase	38% in 3 months	16% in 12 months

*Many studies of saw palmetto extract lasted fewer than 90 days. Final measurements were calculated as 90-day measurements.
**There are no long-term studies of saw palmetto extract, yet its effect at three months is obviously superior to the effect of Proscar.

obstruction due to an enlarged prostate). The data in Table 4.1 are based on pooled data from clinical studies.

Clearly, saw palmetto extract is superior to Proscar. It is also significantly less expensive—it is at least one-fourth the price. The standard dosage of the fat-soluble saw palmetto extract standardized to contain 85% to 95% fatty acids and sterols is 160 milligrams, twice daily. For best results, make sure you are using the right extract at the right dosage. Detailed toxicology studies of the extract have been carried out on mice, rats, and dogs. None indicates that the extract has toxic effects. No significant side effects have ever been reported in the clinical trials of the extract or after saw palmetto berry ingestion.

Use of Flower Pollen Extract

The flower pollen extract known by the product name Cernilton has been used in Europe to treat prostatitis and BPH for more than 25 years.[22] (Cernilton is a product of A. B. Cernelle of Sweden.) Several double-blind clinical studies show it to be quite effective in the treatment of prostatitis due to inflammation or infection.[23,24] The extract exerts some anti-inflammatory action and produces a contractile effect on the bladder. Simultaneously, it relaxes the urethra. Cernilton and similar products are available in health food stores. Although these products are perhaps best suited for the treatment of prostatitis, they can also be helpful in treating BPH. The standard dosage of Cernilton and similar products is 2 tablets, three times daily.

Use of Pygeum africanum Extract

Another herbal medicine useful in various prostate disorders is made from the bark of *Pygeum africanum*. Pygeum is an evergreen tree native to Africa whose bark has historically been used in the treatment of urinary tract disorders. The major active components of the bark are fat-soluble sterols and fatty acids. Virtually all the research on pygeum has featured a pygeum extract standardized to contain 14% triterpenes, including beta-sitosterol and 0.5% *n*-docosanol. This extract has been extensively studied, in animal studies and clinical trials in humans.

The primary target organ for pygeum's effects in males is the prostate. The various fat-soluble components of pygeum appear to exert different, yet complementary, effects on BPH. In addition, pygeum has been shown to enhance the secretions of the prostate and bulbourethral glands, both in terms of quantity and quality.

Numerous clinical trials in over 600 patients have demonstrated that pygeum extract is effective in reducing the symptoms and clinical signs of BPH, especially in early cases.[25-30] However, in a double-blind study that compared the effects of pygeum extract with those of the extract of saw palmetto, the saw palmetto extract produced a greater reduction of symptoms and was better tolerated.[31] In addition, the effects on objective parameters, especially urine flow rate and residual urine content, were better in the clinical studies of saw palmetto. However, there may be circumstances where pygeum is more effective than saw palmetto. For example, saw palmetto has not been shown to produce some of the effects that pygeum has produced on prostate secretion. Of course, as the two extracts have somewhat overlapping mechanisms of action, they can be used in combination.

Pygeum may be effective in improving fertility in cases where diminished prostatic secretion plays a significant role. Pygeum can increase prostatic secretions and improve the composition of the seminal fluid.[32-34] Specifically, pygeum administration to men with decreased prostatic secretion has led to increased levels of total seminal fluid plus increases in enzymes and protein.

What is more, in a double-blind clinical trial, pygeum extract showed an ability to help patients with BPH or prostatitis improve their capacity to achieve an erection.[35] BPH and prostatitis are often associated with erectile dysfunction and other sexual disturbances. Presumably, by improving the underlying condition, pygeum can improve sexual function.

The dosage of the fat-soluble extract of *Pygeum africanum* standardized to contain 14% triterpenes (including beta-sitosterol and 0.5% *n*-docosanol) is 100 to 200 milligrams per day, in divided doses.

Use of Hot Sitz Baths

Hot sitz baths can be beneficial in the treatment of prostate disorders. To take a sitz bath is to partially immerse the pelvic region in water. Although a sitz bath is more easily taken in a specially constructed tub, a regular bathtub can suffice. The water should be from 105 degrees to 115 degrees Fahrenheit. Immerse the pelvic region for 3 to 10 minutes, then sponge the pelvic area with cool water. The primary effect of a sitz bath is relaxation and the opening of the urinary passageway. *Hot sitz baths are not indicated in cases of acute inflammation or infection of the prostate or those involving fertility problems due to high scrotal temperature.*

Chapter Summary

Prostate disorders, including BPH and prostate cancer, are quite common. Because symptoms of BPH and prostate cancer are similar, a physician must perform the proper measures to make a sound diagnosis. The best treatment of prostate cancer is prevention by consuming a diet that is low in sugar, animal fat and protein, and high in plant foods (especially sources of carotenes).

In the prevention and treatment of BPH and prostatitis, important dietary factors include avoidance of pesticides, synthetic hormones, and beer, and adequate intake and absorption of zinc, essential fatty acids, and vitamin B6. BPH patients who need more than dietary support should use the extract of saw palmetto berries. Prostatitis patients should use flower pollen extract.

5

Male Genitourinary Tract Infections

Infections in the male genitourinary tract—including infections of the epididymis, seminal vesicles, prostate, bladder, and urethra—are thought to play a major role in many cases of infertility as well as reduced sexual vitality.[1] The exact extent of the role they play is largely unknown because of the lack of suitable diagnostic criteria, coupled with the fact that many infections are without symptoms. In the absence of other clinical findings, the presence of antisperm antibodies is a good indicator of a chronic infection.

A comprehensive exam by a physician is essential if you are experiencing any symptoms of an infection. If there is any discharge from the penis, pain or burning sensation with urination or ejaculation, pain in the scrotum or pelvic region, or the appearance of anything abnormal on your genitalia, *consult a physician immediately.*

Chlamydia

There are a wide number of bacteria, viruses, and other organisms that can infect the male genitourinary system. It is beyond the scope of this book to discuss every type of infection; therefore, the discussion will be limited to *Chlamydia trachomatis.* This organism has some characteristics of a virus and some characteristics of a bacteria. It's like a virus in that it is a parasite that lives within human cells, but its structure resembles that of a bacterium.

Chlamydia is now recognized as the most common as well as the most serious male genitourinary tract infection.[1] Chlamydia is considered a sexually transmitted disease. In women, chlamydia infection can lead to pelvic inflammatory disease (PID) and scarring of the fallopian tubes. Chlamydia infection accounts for a large number of cases of female infertility.

In men, chlamydia infection can lead to equally disabling effects. It is the major cause of acute nonbacterial prostatitis and urethritis. The typical symptom is pain or a burning sensation upon urination or ejaculation. More serious is chlamydia infection of the epididymis and vas deferens. The resultant damage to these organs parallels the tubal damage in women. Serious scarring and blockage can occur. During an acute chlamydia infection, antibiotics are essential. Chlamydia is sensitive to tetracyclines and erythromycin. Unfortunately, because chlamydia lives within human cells, it may be difficult to totally eradicate the organism with antibiotics alone.

Although acute chlamydial infections are usually associated with severe pain, chronic infections of the urethra, seminal vesicles, or prostate can persist with few or no symptoms. Chlamydia is thought to play a role in some cases of male infertility. It is estimated that 28% to 71% of infertile men have evidence of a chlamydial infection.[1]

Because of the possible link between chlamydia and low sperm counts, several double-blind studies have researched the effects of antibiotics on sperm counts. These studies have not been too positive; very little improvements in sperm count or sperm quality were noted. However, there have been isolated cases of tremendous increases in sperm counts and sperm quality after antibiotic treatment. If electing this form of treatment, both partners should take the antibiotic. I do not recommend an antibiotic as an indiscriminate male fertility aid. Use antibiotics only if there is reason to believe a chronic infection is present and after you have followed, for at least 3 months, the recommendations given in Chapter 4 and those given in this chapter. The presence of antisperm antibodies may be a clue to a chronic chlamydia infection. In the absence of a positive culture, rectal ultrasonography and the detection of antibodies directed against chlamydia can confirm the diagnosis.

The Natural Approach to Male Genitourinary Tract Infections

The primary goal in the natural approach to treating male genitourinary tract infections is enhancing normal protective measures. Specifically, this refers to:

- Enhancing the flow of urine by achieving and maintaining proper hydration
- Promoting a pH that will inhibit the growth of the organism
- Preventing bacterial adherence to the endothelial cells of the urethra and bladder
- Making sure that adequate zinc levels are attained for the production of zinc-containing antimicrobial compounds secreted by the prostate
- Enhancing the immune system

In addition, several plant-based medicines can be employed, including the flower pollen extract described in Chapter 4.

The measures discussed in this chapter are of a general nature and can be used to treat virtually any genitourinary tract infection, including chlamydia. It is imperative that these measures be part of a *supervised* treatment plan. Do not attempt to treat an acute or even chronic infection without the supervision of a trained health care professional.

Increased Urine Flow

Increasing urine flow can be easily achieved by increasing the amount of liquids consumed. Ideally, the liquids consumed should be in the form of pure water, fresh juices diluted with an equal amount of water, and herbal teas. Drink at least 64 ounces of liquids from this group, with at least half of this amount being water. Avoid soft drinks, concentrated fruit drinks, coffee, and alcoholic beverages.

Of particular benefit in the treatment of urinary tract infections are cranberries and cranberry juice. Both have been used to treat bladder infections and have been shown to be quite effective in several clinical studies.[2-5] In one study, 16 ounces of cranberry juice per day produced beneficial effects in 73% of the subjects (44 females and 16 males) with active urinary tract infections.[3] Furthermore, withdrawal of the cranberry juice in the people who benefited resulted in recurrence of bladder infection in 61%.

Many people believe the action of cranberry juice is due to acidification of the urine and the antibacterial effects of a cranberry component, hippuric acid.[6,7] However these are probably not the major mechanisms of action. In order to acidify the urine, a patient would have to drink at least 1 quart of cranberry juice at one sitting.[6] In addition, the concentration of hippuric acid in the urine as a result of drinking cranberry juice is not sufficient to inhibit bacteria.[6,7]

In the treatment of bladder infection, patients benefited from drinking only 16 ounces of cranberry juice per day. These data indicate that a mechanism other than acidification is at work.

Recent studies have shown that components in cranberry juice reduce the ability of *Escherichia coli* bacteria to stick to the lining of the bladder and urethra.[8,9] For bacteria to infect, they must first adhere to the mucosa. By interfering with adherence, cranberry juice greatly reduces the likelihood of infection and helps the body fight off infection. This is the most likely explanation of the positive effects of cranberry juice on bladder infections.

One study of seven juices (cranberry, blueberry, grapefruit, guava, mango, orange, and pineapple) showed that only cranberry and blueberry contained the inhibitors that reduced adherence.[9] Blueberry juice is a suitable alternative to cranberry juice in the treatment of bladder infections.

Note, however, that most cranberry juices on the market contain one-third cranberry juice mixed with water and sugar. Since sugar has such a detrimental effect on the immune system,[10-12] use of sweetened cranberry juice cannot be recommended. Fresh cranberry juice (sweetened with apple or grape juice) or blueberry juice is preferred. Cranberry extracts are also available commercially, in pill form.

Acidification or Alkalinization?

Although many practitioners believe acidifying the urine is the best approach in addressing a urinary tract infection, several arguments can be made for alkalinizing the urine. First of all, it is often very difficult to acidify the urine. At commonly prescribed doses, popular urine-acidification methods, such as using ascorbic acid supplements and drinking cranberry juice, have very little effect on pH.

The best argument for alkalinizing the urine is that it seems more effective than acidifying. The best method for alkalinizing the urine appears to be the use of citrate salts—potassium citrate or sodium citrate, for example. These salts are rapidly absorbed and metabolized without affecting gastric pH or producing a laxative effect. They are excreted partly as carbonate, thus raising the pH of the urine.

Because, at typical dosages, they do no harm and often do good, potassium citrate and/or sodium citrate have long been prescribed as therapies to use until the results of a urine culture are available. There are some clinical studies to support this practice. For example, in one study, women with symptoms of a urinary tract infection were given a 4-gram dose of sodium citrate every 8 hours for 48 hours.[13] Of the 64 women evaluated, 80% of the women experienced relief of symptoms, 12% noticed a lessening of symptoms, and 91.8% of the women rated the treatment as acceptable. Of the 64 women, 19 had positive bacterial cultures. More variation in response to treatment occurred in the groups with proven bacterial infection and urethral pain (7 of 10) and painful or difficult urination (13 of 18) than in those complaining of urinary frequency (9 of 17) and urgency (6 of 13). These results were very similar to those of a previous study, which demonstrated significant symptomatic relief in 80% of the 159 women whose bacterial cultures were negative.[14]

One more possible advantage lies in alkalizing, rather than acidifying, the urine. Many of the herbs used to treat urinary tract infections, such as goldenseal and uva-ursi, contain antibacterial components that work most effectively in an alkaline environment.

Plant-Based Medicines

Many plants have been used through the centuries in the treatment of male genitourinary tract infections. In my opinion, the three best are uva-ursi, goldenseal, and bromelain.

Using Uva-Ursi   Also known as bearberry and upland cranberry, uva-ursi (*Arctostaphylos uva-ursi*) is a small evergreen shrub found in the northern United States and in Europe. Uva-ursi has a long history of use for its diuretic and antiseptic properties. Its major antiseptic component in regard to the urinary tract is arbutin, which typically composes 7% to 9% of the leaves. Arbutin is an effective urinary tract antiseptic, but the effect of arbutin is less than that of the total uva-ursi plant.[14] Crude plants or their extracts are often much more effective medicinally than the isolated active constituent. This appears to be the case with uva-ursi and arbutin.

The arbutin molecule must be absorbed intact from the intestine. When arbutin is given alone, bacteria in the intestine break down much of the arbutin before it is absorbed. If the whole plant is given, there are components in the plant that prevent this breakdown. For arbutin to be active, it must be converted to another compound, hydroquinone, in the urinary tract. If the whole plant or crude extract is given, the net effect is an increase in the amount of arbutin that is converted to hydroquinone.

Uva-ursi extracts are especially active against *E. coli* bacteria.[15] The activity of arbutin as an antibiotic in the urinary tract is dependent on alkaline urine.[16] This suggests another reason why the whole plant is of more value than the isolated compound: The nonarbutin components of uva-ursi alkalinize the urine. Daily dosages for various forms of uva-ursi follow.

Dried leaves or as an infusion (tea)	1.5 to 4.0 grams (1 to 2 teaspoons)
Freeze-dried leaves	500 to 1,000 milligrams
Tincture (1:5)	4 to 6 milliliters (1 to 1½ teaspoons)

| Fluid extract (1:1) | 0.5 to 2.0 milliliters (¼ to ½ teaspoon) |
| Powdered solid extract (10% arbutin content) | 250 to 500 milligrams |

Using Goldenseal   Native Americans used goldenseal (*Hydrastis canadensis*) extensively as a medication and clothing dye. Its medicinal use resulted from its ability to soothe the mucous membranes that line the respiratory, digestive, and genitourinary tracts, especially in inflammatory conditions induced by allergy or infection.

The medicinal value of goldenseal (as well as barberry and Oregon grape root) is thought to be due to its high content of alkaloids, of which berberine has been the most widely studied. Perhaps the most celebrated of berberine's effects has been its broad spectrum of antibiotic activity. Berberine has shown antimicrobial activity against chlamydia as well as many disease-causing bacteria, protozoa, and fungi.[16-19]

Its action against some of these organisms is actually stronger than that of antibiotics commonly used. In addition, researchers have shown that berberine prevents the adherence of bacteria to human cells.[20] By blocking adherence, infection is thwarted. Berberine also activates the immune system, particularly macrophages.[21] These cells are responsible for engulfing and destroying bacteria, viruses, tumor cells, and other particulate matter.

Several clinical studies have shown that berberine can be highly successful in the treatment of acute diarrhea.[22-24] Berberine has been found effective against diarrheas caused by *E. coli* (traveler's diarrhea), *Shigella dysenteriae* (shigellosis), *Salmonella paratyphi* (food poisoning), *Giardia lamblia* (giardiasis), and *Vibrio cholerae* (cholera). Presumably, goldenseal would have effects similar to those of berberine.

In addition, berberine has inhibited *Chlamydia trachomatis* in clinical trials involving patients with trachoma, an infectious eye disease due to *C. trachomatis*.[25,26] One study compared berberine (0.2%) to the drug sulfacetamide (20.0% solution). Sulfacetamide caused the most improvement initially, but the cultures from the eyes of all patients receiving sulfacetamide were still positive for chlamydia. The patients receiving sulfacetamide had a high rate of symptom recurrence. In contrast, patients treated with the berberine solution showed very mild eye symptoms, which disappeared more gradually, but their cultures were always negative for chlamydia. These patients did not suffer relapse even one year after treatment, which suggests that berberine is probably more curative for trachoma than sulfacetamide, even though the concentration of berberine was 100 times less than the concentration of sulfacetamide.

Berberine's effect in trachoma is believed to be due to stimulation of some host defense mechanism rather than on a direct action against chlamydia. The impressive clinical results in regard to trachoma, along with the other effects of berberine, indicate that it may be useful in chlamydial genitourinary tract infections.

For best results, goldenseal extracts standardized for berberine content are preferred. For urinary tract infections, I recommend that goldenseal be used in conjunction with bromelain (see the next section). Here are the three-times-a-day dosages for various forms of goldenseal:

Dried root or as an infusion (tea)	2 to 4 grams (1½ to 2 teaspoons)
Tincture (1:5)	6 to 12 milliliters (1½ to 3 teaspoons)
Fluid extract (1:1)	1 to 2 milliliters (¼ to ½ teaspoon)

Solid (powdered dry)   250 to 500 milligrams
extract (4:1 or 8% to
12% alkaloid content)

Using Bromelain   A mixture of enzymes from pineapple, bromelain was introduced as a medicinal agent in 1957. Since that time, over 200 scientific papers on its therapeutic applications have appeared in the medical literature.[16,27] In these scientific studies bromelain exerted a wide variety of beneficial effects, including reduction of inflammation in cases of arthritis, sports injury, or trauma, and prevention of swelling (edema) after trauma or surgery.

Several mechanisms may account for bromelain's anti-inflammatory effects, including the inhibition of pro-inflammatory compounds. Bromelain's anti-inflammatory action may make it useful in treating chronic inflammation of the genitourinary tract, but there is another reason why I like to recommend bromelain.

Clinical studies show that bromelain increases serum levels of a variety of antibiotics (for example, amoxicillin, tetracycline, and penicillin) in many different body fluids and tissues (for example, cerebral spinal fluid, sputum, mucus, blood, and urine, and in the uterus, uterine tubes, ovaries, gallbladder, appendix, and epithelial tissue).[28-30] In addition, researchers concluded that bromelain itself was as effective as antibiotics in treating a variety of infectious processes. These included pneumonia, perirectal abscesses, skin infections, pyelonephritis (kidney disease), and bronchitis.[27,30]

Bromelain may have the same effects on berberine that it has on the antibiotics. If you are taking an antibiotic for a male genitourinary infection, take bromelain with your medication.

The standard dosage of bromelain is based on its milk clotting unit (mcu) activity. The most beneficial range of activity appears to be 1,800 to 2,000 mcu. The dosage to achieve this range is 400 to 500 milligrams, three times daily, on an empty stomach.

Chapter Summary

Infections of the male genitourinary tract may be a cause of decreased sexual vitality and infertility. Chlamydia is emerging as a major cause of infection, and it has serious consequences. Natural measures for treatment include increasing urine flow; alkalinizing the urine; and using plant-based medicines such as uva-ursi, goldenseal, and bromelain.

6

Eating for Virility

Nutrition is the key to maintaining or attaining virility. The goals of eating for virility are:

- Supplying key nutrients required for normal sexual function
- Eating a diet that keeps cholesterol and triglyceride levels in the proper range
- Consuming a diet that lowers the risk of prostate cancer

There is little debate that a healthy diet must be rich in whole "natural" (unprocessed) foods. Of particular importance are plant foods: fruits, vegetables, grains, beans, seeds, and nuts. These foods not only contain valuable nutrients, but they also provide dietary fiber and other food compounds that have remarkable health-promoting properties.

My book *The Healing Power of Foods* contains extensive information on what the human being is designed to eat, what each food contains in terms of nutritional and medicinal qualities, what foods should be consumed for specific health conditions, and detailed recommendations on constructing a healthful diet by using the Healthy Exchange System.[1] The Healthy Exchange System is based on seven lists:

List 1   Vegetables

List 2   Fruits

List 3   Breads, cereals, and starchy vegetables

List 4   Legumes

List 5   Fats and oils

List 6   Milk

List 7   Meats, fish, cheese, and eggs

Lists 6 and 7—the milk and meat lists—are optional. All food portions within each list provide approximately the same calories, proteins, fats, and carbohydrates. (The fact that the servings are equal in this sense gives rise to the term *exchange*—any item in one list can be exchanged for any item in the same list.) To use the Healthy Exchange System, you begin by determining whether you will be a vegan (someone who does not consume meat or dairy products) or an omnivore (someone who eats animal and vegetable substances). Then you calculate how many calories you need each day to maintain yourself in a healthful way. (You do this by determining your body frame size.) Once you know how many calories you should be consuming, you turn to the diets of the Healthy Exchange System. These are "menus" that tell you how many servings from each Healthy Exchange List you should eat to consume the number of daily calories appropriate for you.

To simplify matters, I will assume that you need 2,500 calories each day. (If you would like to construct an eating program that is more personal, I urge you to do so; see *The*

Healing Power of Foods.) The list that follows shows how many servings from each Healthy Exchange List you need to eat each day to attain optimal nutrition if you are a vegan.

2,500-Calorie Vegan Diet

List 1 (vegetables)	8 servings
List 2 (fruits)	3 servings
List 3 (breads, cereals, and starchy vegetables)	16 servings
List 4 (legumes)	5 servings
List 5 (fats and oils)	9 servings

This diet results in an intake of approximately 2,500 calories, of which 65% are derived from complex carbohydrates (cereals, fruits, and vegetables) and naturally occurring sugars, 19% from fats, and 16% from proteins. The protein intake is entirely from plant sources, but still provides approximately 101 grams of protein, an amount well above the recommended daily allowance for someone requiring 2,500 calories. At least one-half of the fat servings should be from nuts, seeds, and other whole foods from list 5, the fat exchange list. The dietary fiber intake is 31 to 74.5 grams. The list that follows summarizes this information.

Percentage of calories as carbohydrates: 65%

Percentage of calories as fats: 19%

Percentage of calories as protein: 16%

Protein content: 101 grams

Dietary fiber content: 31 to 74.5 grams

The list that follows shows how many servings from each Healthy Exchange List you should eat if you are an omnivore.

2,500-Calorie Omnivore Diet

List 1 (vegetables)	8 servings
List 2 (fruits)	3½ servings
List 3 (breads, cereals, and starchy vegetables)	17 servings
List 4 (legumes)	2 servings
List 5 (fats and oils)	8 servings
List 6 (milk)	1 serving
List 7 (meats, fish, cheese, and eggs)	3 servings

Percentage of calories as carbohydrates: 66%

Percentage of calories as fats: 18%

Percentage of calories as protein: 16%

Protein content: 102 grams (80% from plant sources)

Dietary fiber content: 40.5 to 116.5 grams

In the next seven sections, you will learn about the foods in each list and how they can help you. In each section, the appropriate exchange list appears. From these lists, each day, you will choose foods to meet the serving requirements defined by your diet.

List 1: Vegetables

Vegetables provide the broadest range of nutrients of any food class. They are rich sources of vitamins, minerals, carbohydrates, and proteins. The little fat they contain is in the form of essential fatty acids. In addition, vegetables provide high quantities of other valuable health-promoting substances, especially carotenes (substances that can be converted into vitamin A) and fiber. In Latin, the word *vegetable* means to enliven or animate. Vegetables give us life. More and more evidence is accumulating that shows that vegetables can prevent as well as treat many diseases.

Vegetables should play a major role in the diet. The U.S. National Academy of Science, the U.S. Department of Health and Human Services, and the National Cancer Institute recommend that Americans consume a minimum of 3 to 5 servings of vegetables per day.[2] I recommend 8 servings per day.

The best way to consume many vegetables is in their fresh, raw form. In this form, many of their nutrients and health-promoting compounds are provided in much higher concentrations than in processed vegetables. Drinking fresh vegetable juice is an excellent way to make sure you are achieving your daily quota of vegetables.

When cooking vegetables, be sure not to overcook them. Overcooking will not only result in the loss of important nutrients, it will alter the flavor. Light steaming, baking, and quick stir-frying are the best ways to cook vegetables. Do not boil vegetables; most of the nutrients will be left in the water. The only exception to this rule is soup making. Since the liquid used for boiling the vegetables is the soup itself, and you will consume the soup, boiling soup vegetables is fine. If, for soup or other dishes, fresh vegetables are not available, frozen vegetables are preferred over their canned counterparts.

Although pickled vegetables are quite popular, they may not be healthful choices. Not only are they high in salt, they may also be high in cancer-causing compounds. Several population studies in China have suggested an association between consumption of pickled vegetables and cancer of the esophagus.[3] The harmful substances in pickled vegetables are *N*-nitroso compounds. Once ingested, these compounds can form potent cancer-causing nitrosamines.

Vegetables are fantastic "diet" foods because they are very high in nutritional value but low in calories. In list 1 you will notice a category for "free" vegetables. These vegetables are termed free because you can eat them in any amount desired; the calories they contain will be offset by the number of calories your body will burn to digest them. If you are trying to lose weight, these foods are especially valuable because they will help to keep you feeling satisfied between meals.

Vegetables
Vegans: Choose 8 servings from list 1.
Omnivores: Choose 8 servings from list 1.

Measured-serving vegetables
Unless otherwise noted, 1 serving consists of 1 cup of cooked vegetable or fresh vegetable juice or 2 cups of raw vegetable.

Artichoke (1 medium)

Asparagus

Bean sprouts

Beets

Broccoli

Brussels sprouts

Carrots

Cauliflower

Eggplant

Greens

    Beet

    Chard

    Collard

    Dandelion

    Kale

    Mustard

    Spinach

    Turnip

Mushrooms
Okra
Onions
Rhubarb
Rutabaga
Sauerkraut
String beans, green or yellow
Summer squash
Tomatoes, tomato juice, vegetable juice cocktail
Zucchini

Free vegetables
Eat as many of the following items as you wish.

Alfalfa sprouts
Bell peppers
Bok choy
Cabbage
Celery
Chicory
Chinese cabbage
Cucumber
Endive
Escarole
Lettuce
Parsley
Radishes
Spinach
Turnips
Watercress

List 2: Fruits

Fruits are excellent sources of many vital antioxidants, such as vitamin C, carotenes, and flavonoids. However, fruits are not as beneficial as vegetables, because they tend to be higher in calories. That is why vegetables are favored over fruits. Nonetheless, regular fruit consumption has been shown to offer significant protection against many chronic degenerative diseases, including cancer, heart disease, cataracts, and stroke.[1]

Since fruits contain a fair amount of natural fruit sugar, or fructose, most responsible eating programs limit intake to no more than 4 servings of fruit or two 8-ounce glasses of fresh fruit juice per day. Fruits make excellent snacks because fructose is absorbed slowly into the bloodstream, thereby allowing the body time to utilize it.

The Healthy Exchange List for fruit follows. You will note that the list includes a few items made from processed fruit—jams, jellies, and preserves—and a few items that are not fruits at all—honey and sugar. Do not eat more than 1 serving per day of these processed products.

Fruits

Vegans: Choose 3 servings from list 2.

Omnivores: Choose 3½ servings from list 2.

Each of the following items equals 1 serving.

Fresh fruit and fruit-based items

Fresh juice, 1 cup (8 ounces)*

Pasteurized juice, ⅔ cup

Apple, 1 large

Applesauce (unsweetened), 1 cup

Apricots, dried, 8 halves

Apricots, fresh, 4 medium

Banana, 1 medium

Berries,
> Blackberries, 1 cup
>
> Blueberries, 1 cup
>
> Cranberries, 1 cup
>
> Raspberries, 1 cup
>
> Strawberries, 1½ cups

Cherries, 20 large

Dates, 4

Figs, dried, 2

Figs, fresh, 2

Grapefruit, 1

Grapefruit juice, 1 cup

Grapes, 20

Mango, 1 small

Melons
> Cantaloupe, ½ small
>
> Honeydew, ¼ medium
>
> Watermelon, 2 cups

Nectarines, 2 small

Orange, 1 large

Papaya, 1½ cups

Peaches, 2 medium

Persimmons, 2 medium

Pineapple, 1 cup

Plums, 4 medium

Prune juice, ½ cup

Prunes, 4 medium

Raisins, 4 tablespoons

Tangerines, 2 medium

Processed fruit and other products

Eat no more than 1 serving of the following "fruit" foods per day.

Honey, 1 tablespoon

Jams, jellies, preserves, 1 tablespoon

Sugar, 1 tablespoon

*Although 1 cup of most juices equals 1 serving, prune juice is an exception; consult the alphabetized portion of the list.

List 3: Breads, Cereals, and Starchy Vegetables

Breads, cereals, and starchy vegetables are classified as complex carbohydrates. Complex carbohydrates are made up of long chains of simple carbohydrates or sugars. This means the human body has to digest, or break down, the large sugar chains into simple sugars. Therefore, the sugar from complex carbohydrates enters the bloodstream slowly. This means a relatively stable blood sugar level and appetite.

Complex carbohydrates—breads, cereals, and starchy vegetables—are higher in fiber and nutrients and lower in calories than simple-sugar items such as cakes and candies. Choose whole-grain products (whole-grain breads, whole-grain flour products, brown rice, and the like) over their processed counterparts (white bread, white-flour products, white rice, and so on). Whole grains are a major source of complex carbohydrates, dietary fiber, minerals, and B vitamins. The protein content and quality of whole grains is greater than that of refined grains. Diets rich in whole grains guard against chronic degenerative diseases. Whole-grain diets are especially significant in the prevention of cancer, heart disease, diabetes, varicose veins, and diseases of the colon (colon cancer, inflammatory bowel disease, hemorrhoids, and diverticulitis).[2]

Whole grains can be used as breakfast cereals, side dishes, or casseroles or as part of a dinner entrée. Whole-grain recipes appear later in this chapter. Another of my books, *The Healing Power of Foods Cookbook,* also contains whole-grain recipes.

Note that some of the prepared foods included in the list of breads, cereals, and starchy vegetables constitute more than 1 serving.

Breads, Cereals, and Starchy Vegetables

Vegans: Choose 16 servings from list 3.
Omnivores: Choose 17 servings from list 3.
Each of the following items equals 1 serving.

Breads

Bagel, small, ½

Dinner roll, 1

Dried bread crumbs, 3 tablespoons

English muffin, small, ½

Tortilla (6 inch), 1

Whole wheat, rye, or pumpernickel, 1 slice

Cereals

Bran flakes, ½ cup

Cornmeal (dry), 2 tablespoons

Flour, 2½ tablespoons

Grits (cooked), ½ cup

Pasta (cooked), ½ cup

Porridge (cooked cereal), ½ cup

Puffed cereal (unsweetened), 1 cup

Rice or barley (cooked), ½ cup

Unpuffed, unsweetened cereal, ¾ cup

Wheat germ, ¼ cup

Crackers

Arrowroot, 3

Graham (2½-inch squares), 2

Matzo (4 by 6 inches), ½

Rye wafers (2 by 3½ inches), 3

Saltine, 6

Starchy vegetables

Corn, kernels, ⅓ cup

Corn on the cob, 1 small cob

Parsnips, ⅔ cup

Potato, mashed, ½ cup

Potato, white, 1 small

Squash (winter, acorn, or butternut), ½ cup

Yam or sweet potato, ¼ cup

Prepared foods

Each of the following items equals 1 "bread" serving, but you must omit 1 or more fat servings to maintain the nutrition balance of your diet.

Biscuit, 2-inch diameter, 1 (omit 1 fat serving)

Corn bread, 2 by 2 by 1 inch, 1 (omit 1 fat serving)

French fries, 2 to 3 inches long, 8 (omit 1 fat serving)

Muffin, small, 1 (omit 1 fat serving)

Pancake, 5 by ½ inch, 1 (omit 1 fat serving)

Potato or corn chips, 15 (omit 2 fat servings)

Waffle, 5 by ½ inch, 1 (omit 1 fat serving)

List 4: Legumes

According to the dictionary, a legume is a plant that produces a pod that splits on both sides. Of the common human foods, beans, peas, lentils, and peanuts are legumes. The legume category also includes alfalfa, clover, acacia, and indigo. The fossil record indicates that legumes are among the oldest cultivated plants; prehistoric peoples domesticated and cultivated certain legumes for food. Today, legumes are a mainstay in most diets of the world. Legumes are second only to grains in supplying calories and protein to the human population. Compared to grains, they supply about the same number of total calories, but usually provide two to four times as much protein.

Legumes are often called the poor people's meat; they might be better known as the healthy people's meat. Although lacking some key amino acids, legumes can be combined with grains to form what is known as a complete protein. Many legumes, especially soybeans, provide impressive health benefits. Diets rich in legumes are being used to lower cholesterol levels, improve blood glucose control in diabetics, and reduce the risk of many cancers. Obviously, legumes are an important part of a healthful diet.

Legumes, as well as most nuts and seeds, are sources of compounds known as phytosterols. These plant compounds are structurally similar to testosterone and other steroid hormones. The cholesterol-lowering effects of phytosterols are well documented.[4] Phytosterols have also been shown to enhance immune functions, inhibit the Epstein-Barr virus, prevent chemically induced cancers in animals, and exhibit numerous anticancer effects.[5] Some researchers think the body may be able to utilize phytosterols in hormone production, although this remains to be proven. Soybeans are especially rich in a phytosterol called beta-sitosterol. A 3½-ounce serving of soybeans provides approximately 90 milligrams of beta-sitosterol. Soy is also a good source of isoflavonoids (see Chapter 3).

Legumes

Vegans: Choose 5 servings from list 4.
Omnivores: Choose 2 servings from list 4.

In this list, ½ cup of each item, cooked or sprouted, equals 1 serving.

Black-eyed peas

Chickpeas

Garbanzo beans

Kidney beans

Lentils

Lima beans

Pinto beans

Soybeans, including tofu (omit 1 fat serving)

Split peas

Other dried beans and peas

List 5: Fats and Oils

Typically, animal fats are solid at room temperature and are referred to as saturated fats; vegetable fats are liquid at room temperature and are referred to as unsaturated fats or oils. Vegetable oils provide the greatest source of the essential fatty acids linoleic acid and linolenic acid. These fatty acids function in our bodies as components of nerve cells, cellular membranes, and hormonelike substances known as prostaglandins. (Prostaglandins stimulate contraction of smooth muscle, lower blood pressure, regulate body temperature and blood clotting, and help control inflammation.) Essential fatty acids are critical to normal sexual function. Also, they lower cholesterol and protect against atherosclerosis.

Although fats are important to human health, too much fat in the diet, especially saturated fat, is linked to numerous cancers, heart disease, and stroke. Most nutrition experts strongly recommend that total daily fat intake be kept below

30% of total daily calories. In addition, they recommend eating at least twice as much unsaturated fat as saturated fat. This recommendation is easy to follow. Simply reduce the amount of animal products in the diet, consume more nuts and seeds, and use natural polyunsaturated oils (such as canola, safflower, soy, and flaxseed) as salad dressings.

Most commercially available salad dressings, as well as those in restaurants, are full of the wrong type of oil. As an alternative to store-bought dressing, make Herb Dressing—the recipe appears later in this chapter. It includes polyunsaturated and therapeutic vegetable oils in a delicious combination.

Definitely avoid margarine. During the manufacture of margarine and shortening, vegetable oils are hydrogenated. This means that a hydrogen molecule is added to the natural unsaturated fatty-acid molecule of a vegetable oil to make it saturated. Hydrogenation changes the liquid vegetable oil to a solid or semisolid.

A number of researchers and nutritionists have been concerned about the health effects of margarine since it was introduced. Although many Americans assume they are doing their body good by consuming margarine instead of butter, they are actually doing harm. Margarine and other hydrogenated vegetable oils not only increase the amount of LDL cholesterol; they lower the amount of protective HDL cholesterol, interfere with essential fatty-acid metabolism, and are suspected of causing certain cancers.[6] If you desire a butterlike spread, use a canola-oil product that is nonhydrogenated.

Perhaps the best foods for restoring male sexual vitality are nuts and seeds. This is not surprising, since nuts and seeds are the vehicles for plant reproduction. Locked inside them is the potential for an entire plant. Nuts and seeds provide excellent human nutrition: They are especially good sources of essential fatty acids, vitamin E, protein, minerals, fiber, and other health-promoting substances.

Because of the high oil content of nuts and seeds, you might suspect that their frequent consumption would increase obesity. But a large population study of 26,473 Americans revealed that those who consumed the most nuts were the least obese. This statistic is quite interesting. A possible explanation is that the nuts produced satiety, a feeling of appetite satisfaction. This study also demonstrated that high nut consumption was associated with comparatively fewer heart attacks (both fatal and nonfatal).[7]

A recent study was designed to explore the effect of nuts against heart disease. The results, published in the prestigious *New England Journal of Medicine,* showed that, in men with normal blood lipid levels, walnut consumption lowered total cholesterol 12.4%, reduced LDL cholesterol 16.3%, and decreased triglyceride levels 8.3%.[8] Presumably, other nuts exert similar effects on blood lipids. The beneficial effects are thought to be due to the oils in nuts.

Many physicians use flaxseed oil, in combination with evening primrose and black currant oils, for medicinal purposes. Their patients may realize better results by consuming whole nuts and seeds. The oil in fresh nuts and seeds is less likely to be rancid and the whole nut or seed contains many other vital substances in addition to the oil.

In general, nuts and seeds, due to their high oil content, are best purchased and stored in their shells. The shell is a natural protector against light and air, which promote damage by free radicals. Make sure the shells are free from splits, cracks, stains, holes, or other surface imperfections. Do not eat or use moldy nuts or seeds; eating them may not be safe. Also avoid limp, rubbery, dark, or shriveled nutmeats. Store nuts and seeds, in their shells, in a cool, dry environment. If whole nuts and seeds are unavailable, store nutmeats and shell-less seeds in airtight containers in the refrigerator or freezer. Crushed and slivered nuts and nut pieces are the nut products that are most often rancid. Prepare your own nutmeats from whole nuts. Try to eat at least 2 servings of nuts per day.

Fats and Oils

Vegans: Choose 9 servings from list 5.
Omnivores: Choose 8 servings from list 5.
Each of the following items equals 1 serving.

Mono-unsaturated

Olive oil, 1 teaspoon

Olives, 5 small

Polyunsaturated

Almonds, 10 whole

Avocado (4-inch diameter), 1/8 fruit

Peanuts

    Spanish, 20 whole

    Virginia, 10 whole

Pecans, 2 large

Seeds

    Flax, 1 tablespoon

    Pumpkin, 1 tablespoon

    Sesame, 1 tablespoon

    Sunflower, 1 tablespoon

Vegetable oil

    Canola, 1 teaspoon

    Corn, 1 teaspoon

    Flaxseed, 1 teaspoon

    Safflower, 1 teaspoon

    Soy, 1 teaspoon

    Sunflower, 1 teaspoon

Walnuts, 6 small

Saturated (use sparingly)

Bacon, 1 slice

Butter, 1 teaspoon

Cream, heavy, 1 tablespoon
Cream, light or sour, 2 tablespoons
Cream cheese, 1 tablespoon
Mayonnaise, 1 teaspoon
Salad dressing, 2 teaspoons

List 6: Milk

Is milk for everybody? Definitely not. Many people are allergic to milk or lack the enzymes necessary to digest it. The drinking of cow's milk is a relatively new dietary practice for humans. This may be the reason so many people have difficulty with milk. As for male sexual vitality, cow's milk can be a source of estrogens. What is more, the milk protein known as casein appears to promote athero-sclerosis.[9] Many meal-replacement formulas, including Ultra Slim Fast, contain casein. Casein is also used in glues, molded plastics, and paints. Alternatives to cow's milk and casein-containing formulas are soy milk and soy-based formulas. Unlike casein, soy protein actually lowers cholesterol.[10]

Milk
Vegans: Do not choose from list 6.
Omnivores: Choose 1 serving from list 6.
In each of the following items, one cup equals 1 "milk" serving, but for some items you must omit 1 or more fat servings to maintain the nutrition balance of your diet.

Nonfat milk or yogurt
Nonfat soy milk
2% milk or soy milk (omit 1 fat serving)
Lowfat yogurt (omit 1 fat serving)

Whole milk (omit 2 fat servings)
Yogurt (omit 2 fat servings)

List 7: Meats, Fish, Cheese, and Eggs

When choosing from this list, choose primarily from the lowfat group and remove the skin of poultry. This practice will keep the amount of saturated fat low. List 7 provides high concentrations of certain nutrients difficult to get in an entirely vegetarian diet. It provides the full range of amino acids, vitamin B12, and heme iron. The foods in list 7 are sources of nutrients critical to healthy sexual function. Nonetheless, these foods should be eaten in small amounts; 3 or 4 servings daily provides ample amounts of protein and other nutrients.

In general, you should reduce your intake of animal foods. Cold-water fish—such as salmon, mackerel, and herring—may be exceptions to this recommendation. These fish provide oils known as omega-3 fatty acids. In addition to being critical components of the membranes of the sperm cell, these beneficial oils lower cholesterol and triglyceride levels. The omega-3 fatty acids are being recommended to treat or prevent high cholesterol. They are also being recommended for high blood pressure and other cardiovascular diseases; cancer; autoimmune diseases, such as multiple sclerosis and rheumatoid arthritis; allergies and inflammation; eczema; psoriasis; and many others.[11] The majority of studies of omega-3 fatty acids have utilized fish oils (eicosapentaenoic acid [EPA] and docosahexanoic acid [DHA]). Vegans may be able to derive benefits similar to those offered by fish oils by consuming flaxseed oil. It contains linolenic acid, an omega-3 oil that the body can convert to EPA. Linolenic acid exerts many of the same effects as EPA as well as several others.

A substantial body of evidence documents the relationship between increasing the intake of fish oils and the lowering of blood cholesterol. The question remains, however: Should fish oils be taken as a supplement, or should the dietary intake of fish be increased? In an effort to resolve this question, a recent study of 25 men with high cholesterol levels compared, over a five-week period, the effects of eating fish oil from whole fish versus those of consuming an equivalent amount of oil in a fish-oil supplement.[12] Although total cholesterol levels were unchanged in both groups, both fish and fish-oil supplements lowered triglycerides and raised HDL cholesterol.

However, dietary fish produced some benefits that fish-oil supplements did not. In this study dietary fish oil was more effective than the fish-oil supplement in reducing platelet "stickiness." When platelets adhere to each other, they can form a clot. This clot can get stuck in small arteries and produce a heart attack or stroke. These findings suggest that, though both fish consumption and fish-oil supplements produce desirable effects on lipids and lipoproteins, fish consumption is more effective in improving several other factors involved in cardiovascular disease.

Meats, Fish, Cheese, and Eggs

Vegans: Do not choose from this list.
Omnivores: Choose 3 servings from this list.
Each of the following items equals 1 serving.

Lowfat items

Beef, 1 ounce

Baby beef, chipped beef, chuck, round (bottom, top), rump (all cuts), steak (flank, plate), spareribs, tenderloin plate ribs, tripe

Cottage cheese, lowfat, ¼ cup

Fish, 1 ounce

Lamb, 1 ounce
    Leg, loin (roast/chops), ribs, shank, sirloin, shoulder
Poultry (chicken or turkey without skin), 1 ounce
Veal, 1 ounce
    Cutlet, leg, loin, rib, shank, shoulder

Medium-fat items
For each of the following items, omit ½ fat serving.

Beef, 1 ounce
    Canned corned beef, ground (15% fat), rib eye, round
    (ground commercial)
Cheese, 1 ounce
    Farmer, Mozzarella, Parmesan, ricotta
Eggs, 1
Organ meats, 1 ounce
Peanut butter, 2 tablespoons
Pork, 1 ounce
    Boiled, Boston butt, Canadian bacon, loin (all tender-
    loin), picnic

High-fat items
For each of the following items, omit 2 fat servings.

Beef, 1 ounce
    Brisket, corned beef, ground beef (more than 20%
    fat), hamburger, roasts (rib), steaks (club and rib)
Cheese, cheddar, 1 ounce
Duck or goose, 1 ounce
Lamb, breast, 1 ounce
Pork, 1 ounce
    Country-style ham, deviled ham, ground pork, loin,
    spareribs

Menu Planning

The Healthy Exchange System was created to ensure that you are consuming a diet that provides adequate nutrients in their proper ratio. This chapter has given you the number of servings required from each Healthy Exchange List for a 2,500-calorie-a-day diet. These exchange recommendations will help you a great deal in constructing a daily menu—and so will the recipes you will find in the following pages. For more healthful recipes, see my book *The Healing Power of Foods Cookbook*.

Breakfast

Breakfast is an absolute must. Healthful breakfast choices include whole-grain cereals, muffins, and breads, along with fresh whole fruit or fresh fruit juice. Cereals, both hot and cold, and preferably from whole grains, may be the best food choices for breakfast. The complex carbohydrates in the grains provide sustained energy. What is more, an evaluation of data from the National Health and Nutrition Examination Survey II (a national survey of the nutrition and health practices of Americans) disclosed that blood cholesterol levels are lowest among adults who eat whole-grain cereal for breakfast.[13] Those who consumed other breakfast foods had higher blood cholesterol levels than those who ate whole-grain cereal. Levels were highest among those who typically skipped breakfast.

Thanks to an explosion of marketing information, most Americans are aware of the cholesterol-lowering effects of oats. Since 1963, there have been over 20 major clinical studies examining the effect of oat bran on cholesterol levels.[14] Various oat preparations containing either oat bran or oatmeal have been studied, including cereals, muffins, breads, and entrées. The overwhelming majority of the studies demonstrated a very favorable effect on cholesterol levels. In individuals with high cholesterol levels (above

220 milligrams per deciliter), the consumption of the equivalent of 3 grams of water-soluble oat fiber typically lowered total cholesterol by 8% to 23%. One bowl of ready-to-eat oat bran cereal provides approximately 3 grams of fiber. Although oatmeal's fiber content (7%) is less than that of oat bran (15% to 26%), studies have determined that the polyunsaturated fatty acids from the oatmeal contribute as much to the cholesterol-lowering effects of oats as the fiber content. Although oat bran has a higher fiber content, oatmeal is higher in polyunsaturated fatty acids. This makes oat bran and oatmeal equally effective.

Here are a couple of breakfast suggestions:

Granolalike Breakfast

Makes 4 servings

4	cups rolled oats
4	tablespoons sesame seed (ground)
4	tablespoons sunflower seed (ground)
4	tablespoons flaxseed (ground)
¼	cup fresh apple juice
	Cinnamon to taste
1	cup fresh fruit

In a large bowl, mix oats and ground ingredients. Put ½ cup of oat mixture in a small bowl. Store the bulk of the mixture, covered, in the refrigerator. To the ½ cup of grain mixture, add apple juice and stir. Cover and store overnight in the refrigerator. Add cinnamon and 1 cup fresh fruit; stir together.

Dietary Servings Per Recipe Serving
Fruits: 1
Grains and starches: 2
Fats: 3

Nutrition Information Per Recipe Serving
Calories: 350
Carbohydrate: 55%
Protein: 18%
Fat: 27%
Fiber: 1 gram
Calcium: 94 milligrams

The cinnamon and fruit can also be added the night before.

Apple Carrot Muffins

Makes 12 servings (1 muffin per serving)

2½	cups whole-wheat flour
½	cup soy powder
1	teaspoon baking soda
¼	teaspoon salt
¼	teaspoon nutmeg
¼	teaspoon cinnamon
⅛	cup oil
¾	cup raw honey
1	teaspoon vanilla
½	cup apple, grated
½	cup carrot, grated
	Oil, for greasing tin

In a medium-sized bowl, combine all the dry ingredients. In a large bowl, combine all the liquid ingredients. Stir in the apple and carrot. Add the dry ingredients to the liquid mixture. Preheat oven to 400 degrees F. Oil one muffin tin. Spoon the batter into the cups until they are two-thirds full. Bake until a toothpick stuck in the center of the muffin comes out dry (about 20 minutes).

Dietary Servings Per Recipe Serving
Fruits: 1
Grains and starches: 2
Fats: $1/8$

Nutrition Information Per Recipe Serving
Calories: 220
Carbohydrate: 60%
Protein: 15%
Fat: 25%
Fiber: 4 grams
Calcium: 53 milligrams

An Apple-Carrot Muffin is a great way to start the day, along with a glass of fresh orange juice.

Lunch

Lunch is a fine time to enjoy a healthful bowl of soup, a large salad, and some whole-grain bread. Bean soups and other legume dishes are especially good lunch selections for people with diabetes and blood sugar problems; these selections can improve blood sugar regulation. Legumes are filling, yet low in calories, and provide many nutrients essential for proper sexual function.

Black-Bean Soup

Makes 4 servings

2   teaspoons extra-virgin olive oil *or* canola oil
2   medium red onions, chopped
1   jalapeño chile, minced
2   large garlic cloves, minced

1	teaspoon ground cumin
½	teaspoon chili powder
2	cups water
4	cups cooked black beans
2	tablespoons sour cream (*optional*)

In a medium saucepan, heat olive oil. Add onion and chile. Cook over moderate heat, stirring frequently, until onion begins to brown (about 4 minutes). Stir in garlic. Reduce heat to low and cook, stirring constantly, for 1 minute. Stir in cumin and chili powder. Remove from heat. In a large heavy pot, place the water, beans, and spice mixture. Cook over low heat, stirring occasionally, until beans are hot (about 5 minutes). If a smooth texture is preferred, transfer the soup to a food processor or blender and purée before serving. Top each serving with sour cream.

Dietary Servings Per Recipe Serving
Vegetables: 1
Legumes: 2
Fats: ½

Nutrition Information Per Recipe Serving
Calories: 248
Carbohydrate: 65%
Protein: 19%
Fat: 16%
Fiber: 22 grams
Calcium: 137 milligrams

This soup can be made up to four days ahead. Simply refrigerate it in an airtight container, then reheat it when you're ready.

Herb Dressing

Makes 8 servings (2 tablespoons per serving)

6   tablespoons vegetable oil
2   teaspoons chopped fresh parsley
2   teaspoons chopped fresh chives
2   tablespoons chopped fresh chervil *or* 2 teaspoons
      dried chervil
      Black pepper, to taste
½   cup rice vinegar
2   tablespoons water
3   cloves garlic, minced
2   teaspoons dried mustard

In a blender combine all ingredients. Blend thoroughly.

Snacks

The best snacks are nuts, seeds, fresh fruit, and vegetables.
If you have a sweet tooth, here is a healthful cookie recipe.

Sunflower Power Cookies

Makes 24 servings (1 cookie per serving)

1   cup chopped dried apricots
      Oil, for greasing pan
¼   cup raw honey
1   tablespoon vegetable oil
1   teaspoon vanilla
2   cups rolled oats
1   cup whole-wheat pastry flour

¼   cup toasted wheat germ
½   cup currants *or* raisins
1   tablespoon sunflower seeds
2   tablespoons apple *or* orange juice, if needed

Preheat oven to 350 degrees F. Soak apricots in warm water for 15 minutes. Grease a 13- by 9- by 2-inch baking pan. In a large bowl, mix honey, oil, and vanilla. In a medium bowl, combine oats, flour, and wheat germ. Add flour mixture to wet mixture. Drain apricots. Fold apricots, currants, and sunflower seed into the large bowl, using apple juice to make the batter more pliable if it is too stiff. Press dough into oiled pan. Bake for 20 to 25 minutes. Cool and cut into squares.

Dietary Servings Per Recipe Serving
Fruits: 1
Grains and starches: ½
Fats: ¼

Nutrition Information Per Recipe Serving
Calories: 136
Carbohydrate: 66%
Protein: 8%
Fat: 26%
Fiber: 8 grams
Calcium: 75 milligrams

Kids love these cookies and for good reason—they are delicious. They are also far superior, nutritionally, to store-bought cookies.

Dinner

For dinner, the most healthful meals contain a fresh vegetable salad, a cooked vegetable side dish or bowl of soup, whole grains, and legumes. The whole grains may be provided in bread, pasta, or pizza; as a side dish; or in an entrée. The legumes can be in soups, salads, and main dishes.

Although a varied diet rich in whole grains, vegetables, and legumes can provide optimal levels of protein, many people like to eat meat. The important thing is not to over-consume animal products. Limit your intake to no more than 4 to 6 ounces per day, and choose fish, skinless poultry, and lean cuts rather than fat-ladened choices.

The next recipe provides a complete-protein meal from vegetarian sources.

Mushroom Stroganoff with Tofu

Makes 4 servings

Stroganoff

1	teaspoon canola oil *or* olive oil
½	onion, minced
1	clove garlic, minced (*optional*)
1	pound fresh mushrooms, sliced
4	ounces tofu, cut into 1-inch cubes
1	teaspoon oregano
2	cups cooked brown rice
1	tablespoon toasted slivered almonds
1	tablespoon chopped fresh parsley

Sauce

8	ounces tofu
¼	cup water
2	tablespoons soy sauce
2	tablespoons lemon juice *or* apple cider vinegar
1	clove garlic
1	teaspoon chopped ginger root

Make sauce first. In a large skillet, heat oil. Add onion and garlic; sauté until onion is transparent. Add mushrooms; sauté until they are slightly limp and moisture has evaporated. Remove ingredients from skillet and set them aside. Add tofu cubes to skillet and brown them slightly. Return sautéed ingredients to skillet. Pour sauce over all. Mix well and heat through, stirring. Blend in oregano. Serve over cooked brown rice (½ cup per person) and sprinkle with almonds and parsley.

Sauce. In a blender, combine all ingredients. Blend until very smooth; be sure garlic and ginger root are finely chopped and not left in chunks. Set aside or refrigerate to use later; this improves flavor. Sauce will keep up to 1 week.

Dietary Servings Per Recipe Serving
Vegetables: ½
Grains and starches: 1
Legumes: 1
Fats: ½

Nutrition Information Per Recipe Serving
Calories: 208
Carbohydrate: 56%
Protein: 21%
Fat: 23%
Fiber: 3 grams
Calcium: 160 milligrams

This recipe is a great alternative to Beef Stroganoff.

Chapter Summary

The dietary program presented in this chapter provides optimal nutrition. In addition to providing essential nutrients for proper sexual and reproductive function, the dietary recommendations will lower cholesterol and reduce the risk of heart disease and prostate cancer.

7

Nutritional Supplements

In the last few years, more Americans than ever are taking nutritional supplements. Despite the fact that tremendous scientific evidence supports nutritional supplementation, medical experts have not overwhelmingly endorsed it. Some say diet alone can provide all the nutrition necessary; many others tout the health benefits of supplemental vitamins and minerals. The consumer is left in the middle, trying to figure out which side is right.

First of all, to an extent, both sides are right. What it boils down to is what criteria of "optimal" nutrition are being used. If an expert believes optimal nutrition simply means no obvious signs of nutrient deficiency, his or her answer about whether supplementation is necessary is going to be different from that of an expert who thinks of optimal nutrition as the level of nutrition that will allow a person to function at the highest degree possible, with vitality, energy, and enthusiasm for living. What it comes down to, then, is an argument of philosophy.

Do you believe that health is simply a matter of not being sick? Or do you believe health is much more than this? It is the goal of optimal health that prompts people to take nutritional supplements.

Who Takes Vitamins?

Taking vitamin and mineral supplements has become a way of life for most Americans. Data from the first and second United States Health and Nutrition Examination Survey (HANES I and II), conducted in the 1970s, indicated that almost 35% of the U.S. population between 18 to 74 years of age took vitamin or mineral supplements regularly.[1] During the 1980s and early 1990s, estimates suggest that the number has nearly doubled; now over 70% of Americans take vitamin or mineral supplements.

Although now somewhat outdated, the HANES data demonstrated some interesting facts about supplement users.[1] Perhaps the most interesting was that persons with the highest dietary nutrient intakes are the most likely to take a multiple-vitamin, multiple-mineral supplement. This is extremely significant because it says a great deal about how these individuals define optimal nutrition. They are not using nutritional supplements to bolster a nutrient-poor diet. Instead, they are using supplements as they are truly intended: to supplement a healthful diet.

Here are some other interesting facts from the HANES studies:

- College-educated individuals are much more likely to take a multiple-vitamin, multiple-mineral supplement than those with less education.
- More women take supplements than men do.
- Supplement use is highest in the West and lowest in the South.

- Individuals of normal weight or less are more likely to take supplements than heavier individuals.
- Those who exercise regularly are more likely to take a supplement than those who do not exercise regularly.

The Need for Nutritional Supplementation

Many Americans consume diets inadequate in nutritional value. Their diets are not sufficiently inadequate for nutrient deficiencies to be apparent, however. The term *subclinical deficiency,* or *marginal deficiency,* describes this condition. In many instances, the only clue of a subclinical deficiency is fatigue, lethargy, difficulty in concentration, lack of a feeling of well-being, or some other vague symptom. Diagnosis of subclinical deficiency is an extremely difficult process that involves detailed dietary or laboratory analysis.

Is there evidence to support the contention that subclinical vitamin and mineral deficiencies exist? Definitely yes. During recent years the U.S. government has sponsored a number of comprehensive studies (HANES I and II, Ten State Nutrition Survey, USDA nationwide food consumption studies, to name a few) to determine the nutrition status of the population. These studies have revealed that marginal nutrient deficiencies exist in approximately 50% of the U.S. population. These studies showed that, in regard to some selected nutrients in certain age groups, more than 80% of an age group consumed less than the recommended dietary allowances (RDAs).[2]

These studies indicate that the chances of consuming a diet meeting the RDA for all nutrients is extremely unlikely for most Americans. In other words, though it is theoretically possible for healthy individuals to get all the nutrition they need from foods, the fact is that most Americans do not even come close to meeting all their nutrition needs through diet alone. In an effort to increase their intake of essential nutrients, many Americans look to vitamin and mineral supplements.

A Quick Guide to Vitamin and Mineral Supplementation

Table 7.1 lists recommendations for the daily intake of vitamins and minerals. These recommendations are designed to provide an optimal intake range for maintaining or achieving health. These recommended levels are most easily attained by taking a high-quality multiple-vitamin, multiple-mineral formula and then adding specific nutrients (such as vitamin C, inositol hexaniacinate, vitamin E, or zinc) if there is an increased need for them.

Zinc Supplements

The importance of zinc to male sexual function has been stressed throughout this book. In addition to being important to the sexual system, zinc is critical to virtually every other tissue in the body. Zinc is a component in over 300 enzymes in our bodies. In fact, zinc functions in more enzymatic reactions than any other mineral. Although severe zinc deficiency is very rare in developed countries, many individuals in the United States have marginal zinc deficiency. In addition to impaired sexual function, a marginal zinc deficiency may be reflected by an increased susceptibility to infection, poor wound healing, a decreased sense of taste or smell, or skin disorders.[3]

Optimal zinc levels must be attained if sexual vitality and good health are desired. Many men can benefit by supplementing their healthful diet with zinc. The effectiveness of oral zinc supplementation is dependent on absorption of the ingested zinc. Certain forms of zinc appear to be

Table 7.1 Recommendations for Adult Men, Regarding Daily Intake of Vitamins and Minerals

Vitamins	Daily Supplementation Range
A (retinol)	5,000–10,000 IU*
A (from beta-carotene)	10,000–75,000 IU
D	100–400 IU
E (d-alpha-tocopherol)	400–1,200 IU
K (phytonadione)	60–900 μg**
C (ascorbic acid)	500–9,000 mg
B1 (thiamine)	10–90 mg
B2 (riboflavin)	10–90 mg
Niacin	10–90 mg
Niacinamide	10–30 mg
B6 (pyridoxine)	25–100 mg
Biotin	100–300 μg
Pantothenic acid	25–100 mg
Folic acid	400–1,000 μg
B12	400–1,000 μg
Choline	150–500 mg
Inositol	150–500 mg
Minerals	
Boron	1–2 mg
Calcium	250–500 mg
Chromium	200–400 μg
Copper	1–2 mg
Iodine	50–150 μg
Iron	15 mg
Magnesium	250–500 mg
Manganese	10–15 mg
Molybdenum	10–25 μg
Potassium	200–500 mg
Selenium	100–200 μg
Silica	200–1,000 μg
Vanadium	50–100 μg
Zinc	15–30 mg

*IU = international units
**μg = microgram (one-millionth of a gram)

better absorbed than others. Currently, it appears that zinc picolinate, zinc citrate, and zinc momomethionine are the most absorbable forms.

If you suffer from erectile dysfunction, low sperm count, chronic prostate infection, or benign prostatic hyperplasia, I recommend that—in addition to the regular consumption of foods rich in zinc (particularly pumpkin and sunflower seeds)—you take 45 to 60 milligrams of zinc daily. If you are taking a daily supplement that contains 15 milligrams of zinc, this means you must take an additional 30 to 45 milligrams of zinc each day.

Other Nutritional Supplements

In addition to vitamins and minerals, many other nutritional supplements provide exceptional health benefits. For example, the benefits of carnitine and glandular products containing bovine testicular tissue were described in Chapter 3. Other nutrients that may be important for male sexual function include coenzyme Q10; bee by-products (pollen, royal jelly, and propolis); spirulina, chlorella, and other algae products; wheat and barley grass juice; wheat-germ products; and lecithin. View these products as accessory supplements. Use them in addition to primary recommended supplements rather than as sole therapy. Although they are health-promoting substances, they are not panaceas. In addition, they can be quite costly.

As an example of these accessory supplements, consider royal jelly. Royal jelly is produced by worker bees. Between the 6th and 12th days of the so-called nurse bees' lives, they mix honey and pollen with enzymes in their pharyngeal glands to produce a thick, milky substance—royal jelly— that they feed to the queen bee. That royal jelly is a nutritious food is evident by the queen bee's superior size, astounding ovulation, stamina, and longevity. It contains all the B vitamins, including high concentrations of pantothenic acid (B5) and pyridoxine (B6).

Royal jelly is highly regarded by many health experts for its ability to increase an individual's overall vitality. Its effects supposedly include improved sexual function, although there are no scientific studies to confirm any of these claims. Royal jelly is certainly a nutritious food, but is it worth the relatively high cost? Yes and no. Yes if you can afford it, and no if you can't. If you can afford it, the benefit that you may possibly gain is worth the investment. If you can't afford it, you are probably better off following the dietary recommendations and taking a multiple-vitamin, multiple-mineral formulation.

Chapter Summary

Optimal nutrition is critical if your goal is sexual vitality. Supplementing the diet by taking vitamin and mineral supplements simply makes sense. Think of it as health insurance. In addition to vitamins and minerals, accessory supplements may offer health benefits.

8

Ginseng

There are several different varieties of ginseng: Chinese, Korean, American, and Siberian. I am frequently asked several questions about ginseng, including Is there a difference between the different ginsengs? Does it really matter which one I take? What is the best ginseng? What does ginseng really do? And, can ginseng improve my sex life? I hope to answer these questions and more in this chapter.

What Is the Best Ginseng?

Panax ginseng (Chinese or Korean ginseng) is the most widely used and most extensively studied ginseng. It is generally regarded as the "best" ginseng in that it has the most potent effects. Perhaps the most famous medicinal plant of China, *Panax ginseng* is used alone or in combination with other plants to restore the yang quality. It has also been used as a tonic for its revitalizing properties, especially after a long illness. Ginseng has been used for every condition imaginable, a fact that reflects its broad range of nutritional and medicinal properties.

Panax ginseng contains at least 13 different steroid-like compounds, collectively known as ginsenosides. These compounds are believed to be the most important active constituents of *Panax ginseng*. The usual concentration of ginsenosides in mature ginseng roots is between 1% and 3%. The major ginsenosides are R_0, R_{b1}, R_{b2}, R_{b3}, R_c, R_d, R_e, R_f, 20-gluco-R_f, R_{g1}, and R_{g2}. These differ primarily in their sugar groups, which are attached to the steroid molecule.[1,2]

Ginsenosides R_{b1}, R_{b2}, R_c, R_e, and R_{g1} are present in significant concentrations in Korean ginseng. In contrast, American ginseng (*Panax quinquefolius*) contains, primarily, R_{b1} and R_e. It does not contain R_{b2}; R_f; or, in some instances, R_{g1}. This is extremely important, since R_{b1} and R_{g1} produce different effects. In general, R_{b1} possesses a sedative effect and R_{g1} possesses a stimulatory effect. Since American ginseng is higher in R_{b1} than R_{g1}, its action is much different than that of *Panax ginseng*.

Siberian ginseng (*Eleutherococcus senticosus*) contains no ginsenosides and is not a true ginseng. It can, however, produce many of the same effects as *Panax ginseng*, though it is generally regarded as milder and less potent than the Chinese plant.

Pharmacological Effects of Ginseng

Since the 1950s, a great amount of research has been conducted worldwide to determine whether the properties attributed to *Panax ginseng* belong in the realm of legend or fact. Unfortunately, inconsistent results (due mostly to different procedures in the preparation of extracts, use of different parts of the plant, use of adulterants, and lack of quality control in regard to the ginseng) have made determination of ginseng's true properties difficult. Nonetheless, enough solid research does exist to indicate that *Panax ginseng* possesses activity consistent with its near-legendary status, especially when high-quality extracts, standardized for active constituents, are used.

Adaptogenic Activity

Scientific studies first investigated *Panax ginseng* in regard to its adaptogen qualities. An adaptogen, as defined in 1957 by the Russian pharmacologist I. I. Brekhman, is a substance that (1) must be innocuous and cause minimal disorders in the physiological functions of an organism, (2) must have a nonspecific action (that is, it increases resistance to adverse influences through a wide range of physical, chemical, and biochemical factors), and (3) usually has a normalizing action irrespective of the direction of the pathologic state. According to tradition and scientific evidence, ginseng can cause this kind of equilibrating, tonic, antistress action; therefore, the term *adaptogen* is quite appropriate in describing it.

Siberian ginseng, like *Panax ginseng,* has adaptogenic qualities, but its action is generally regarded as being more gentle than that of *Panax ginseng.* Brekhman discovered the adaptogenic actions of Siberian ginseng as he sought to find an indigenous adaptogen that was more economical than the Chinese plant. American ginseng is also thought to cause adaptogenic activities, although its effects are not well studied.[3]

The adaptogenic qualities of *Panax ginseng,* as well as Siberian ginseng, cause their applications to be varied. From a practical perspective, both can be used as a general tonic, especially for debilitated and feeble individuals. They can also be used to

- Increase feelings of energy
- Increase mental and physical performance

- Prevent the negative effects of stress and enhance the body's response to stress
- Offset some of the negative effects of cortisone
- Enhance liver function
- Protect against radiation damage

Clinical research proves the effectiveness of *Panax ginseng* in all these applications.

Reproductive Effects

Although *Panax ginseng* is claimed as a sexual rejuvenator, human studies supporting this belief do not exist. Ginseng has, however, been shown to promote the growth of the testes, increase sperm formation and testosterone levels, and increase sexual activity and mating behavior in studies with animals.[1,2,4-6] These results seem to support the use of ginseng as a fertility and virility aid.

In regard to the reproductive system, historical use and experimental evidence establish that reasons to use *Panax ginseng* include decreased sperm count; testicular atrophy or hypofunction, including low testosterone secretion; and other organic causes of male infertility. Siberian ginseng is generally used for the same problems. In studies, Siberian ginseng has increased the reproductive capacity and sperm counts of animals.[3]

Antifatigue Activity

High energy levels and sexual vitality go hand in hand. *Panax ginseng* can be used safely to increase energy and fight off fatigue. The mental and physical antifatigue effects of ginseng have been demonstrated in both animal studies and double-blind, clinical trials involving humans. In addition to several Russian studies, which used soldiers and athletes as subjects, other studies support the results of the trials.[7,8] From a practical standpoint, the antifatigue properties of ginseng may be useful whenever fatigue or low vitality is apparent. Athletes, in particular, may derive some benefit from ginseng use.

Antistress Activity

Stress is a term widely used in our fast-paced society. Daily demands often accumulate to the point where it is almost impossible to cope. Job pressures, family arguments, financial pressures, and deadlines are the stressors that probably come to mind first. Actually, a stressor is anything that creates a disturbance, including exposure to heat or cold, environmental toxins, toxins produced by microorganisms, physical trauma, and strong emotional reactions.

As an adaptogen, *Panax ginseng* can enhance the ability to cope with various stressors, both physical and mental. Presumably, this is a result of delaying the alarm phase (fight or flight response) in the classic model of stress. Extensive research suggests that ginseng acts through nervous system control mechanisms to adjust metabolic and functional systems that maintain the body during the challenge of stresses.[1,2] This is very similar to how a thermostat maintains temperature.

In short, *Panax ginseng* causes a balancing effect on the hypothalamic-pituitary-adrenal axis by adjusting metabolic and functional systems that govern hormonal control of homeostasis. Ginseng is indicated when disruption of this axis results in continued stress or the use of corticosteroid drugs.

Cholesterol-Lowering Effects

Atherosclerosis is the major cause of erectile dysfunction. Foremost in the prevention of atherosclerosis is keeping cholesterol and triglyceride levels in the acceptable range. *Panax ginseng* administered to human subjects with elevated cholesterol and triglycerides reduces total serum cholesterol, triglyceride, and fatty-acid levels, while raising the level of HDL cholesterol in the blood.[9] From a clinical perspective, it appears that ginseng may offer some protection against atherosclerotic disease, a factor that further supports its use as a general tonic.

Anticancer Effects

In several animal studies *Panax ginseng* had some effect against cancer. These studies prompted researchers to investigate the effects of ginseng consumption on cancer risk. They interviewed 905 pairs of cases and controls that were matched by age, sex, and date of admission to the Korea Cancer Center Hospital in Seoul.[10] The data revealed that ginseng had a highly statistically significant preventive effect. The effect was greater for ginseng extracts and powders than for fresh sliced ginseng, ginseng juice, or ginseng tea. Researchers noted a dose-response relationship: The higher the intake of ginseng, the lower the risk of cancer.

Dosage

There are many types and grades of ginseng and ginseng extracts. The type and grade depends on the source, age, and parts of the root used, and the methods of preparation. Old, wild, well-formed roots are the most valued; rootlets of cultivated plants are considered the lowest grade. For economic reasons, the majority of ginseng in the American marketplace is derived from the lowest-grade root, diluted with excipients, blended with adulterants, or totally devoid of active constituents (ginsenosides).[11]

High-quality roots and extracts are available, however. These preparations are made from the main root of plants between four and six years of age or extracts that have been standardized for ginsenoside content and ratio to ensure optimum pharmacological effect.

The dosage of *Panax ginseng* depends on the ginsenoside content. If an extract or ginseng preparation contains a high concentration of ginsenosides (and, presumably, other active components), a low dose will suffice.

Currently, there is an almost total lack of quality control in ginseng products marketed in the United States. Independent research and published studies have clearly documented that the ginsenoside content of commercial preparations varies greatly.[11] In fact, the majority of products on the market contain only trace amounts of ginsenosides, and many formulations contain none at all. The lack of quality control has led to several problems, ranging from toxicity reactions (discussed later in this chapter) to absence of medicinal effect. The widespread disregard for quality control in the health food industry has done much to tarnish the reputation of ginseng as well as other important plant-based medicines.

Use standardized ginseng preparations to ensure sufficient ginsenoside content and consistent therapeutic results and to reduce the risk of toxicity. The typical dose (taken one to three times daily) for general tonic effects should contain a saponin content of at least 25 milligrams of ginsenoside R_{g1} with a ratio of R_{g1} to R_{b1} of 2:1. For example, if you have a high-quality *Panax ginseng* root powder containing 5% ginsenosides, the dose would be 500 milligrams; if you have a standardized *Panax ginseng* extract containing an 18% saponin content of ginsenoside R_{g1}, the standard dose would be 150 milligrams. The standard dose for high-quality ginseng root is in the range of 4 to 6 grams, daily.

Siberian ginseng extract is typically standardized according to its eleutheroside-E content (greater than 1%), because there is a correlation between this constituent and the activity of the extract. The typical dosage of Siberian ginseng extract is 100 milligrams, three times daily.

Because each individual's response to ginseng is unique, take care to avoid ginseng toxicity (see the next section). Begin at low doses and increase gradually. The Russian approach for long-term administration is to use ginseng cyclically for a period of 15 to 20 days and then not use ginseng for a two-week interval.

Side Effects

The problem of quality control makes the subject of side effects difficult to address. This dilemma is evident in a 1979 article entitled "Ginseng Abuse Syndrome," which appeared in the *Journal of the American Medical Association*.[12] This article reports a number of side effects, including hypertension, euphoria, nervousness, insomnia, skin eruptions, and morning diarrhea.

Given the extreme variation in quality of ginseng in the American marketplace and the use of various parts of the plant and of adulterants, it is not surprising that side effects were noted. None of the commercial preparations used in the trial had been subjected to controlled analysis. Furthermore, the species of ginseng used included *Panax ginseng, Panax quinquefolius, Eleutherococcus senticosus,* and *Rumex hymenosepalus* in a variety of different forms (roots, capsules, tablets, teas, extracts, cigarettes, chewing gum, and candies).

It is impossible to derive any firm conclusions from the data presented in the JAMA article. The author's final words do, however, seem sensible and appropriate:

An important caveat is that these GAS [ginseng abuse syndrome] effects are neither uniformly negative nor uniformly predictable. Nevertheless, long-term ingestion of large amounts of ginseng should be avoided, as even a panacea can cause problems if abused.

Studies performed on standardized extracts of *Panax ginseng* have demonstrated the absence of side effects as well as no mutagenic or teratogenic effects.[1,2]

Chapter Summary

Panax ginseng is among the world's most popular plant-based medicines. Detailed scientific investigations support the use of ginseng as a general tonic for men and in conditions involving the male reproductive system. These conditions include low sperm count, testicular atrophy or hypofunction, and other organic causes of male infertility.

In addition, ginseng can be used whenever fatigue or lack of energy is apparent, to increase mental and physical performance, to prevent the negative effects of stress and enhance the body's response to stress, to offset the negative effects of cortisone, and to prevent atherosclerosis by lowering cholesterol.

Appendix: Useful Addresses

I hope you have enjoyed this book. If you followed its recommendations and you have not yet experienced benefit, I urge you to consult a naturopath or holistic medical doctor. To find a physician in your area, call or write one of the following addresses:

The American Association of Naturopathic Physicians
P.O. Box 20386
Seattle, WA 98102
(206) 323-7610

The American Holistic Medical Association
4101 Lake Boone Trail, #201
Raleigh, NC 26707
(919) 787-5146

If you are interested in learning more about naturopathic medical schools, write or call the following schools:

Bastyr College of Natural Health Sciences
144 Northeast 54th Street
Seattle, WA 98105
(206) 523-9585

National College of Naturopathic Medicine
11231 Southeast Market Street
Portland, OR 97216
(503) 255-4860

Southwest College of Naturopathic Medicine
6535 East Osborn Road
Scottsdale, AZ 85251
(602) 990-7424

References

Chapter 1: The Male Sexual System

Guyton AC: Textbook of Medical Physiology. Saunders, Philadelphia, 1991.

Chapter 2: Erectile Dysfunction

1. NIH Consensus Conference Panel on Impotence: Impotence. JAMA 270:83–90, 1993.
2. Lerner SE, Melman A, and Christ GJ: A review of erectile dysfunction: New insights and more questions. J Urol 149:1246–55, 1993.
3. Morley JE: Management of impotence. Postgrad Med 93:65–72, 1993.
4. Ornish D, Brown SE, Scherwitz LW, et al.: Can lifestyle changes reverse coronary heart disease? Lancet 336:129–33, 1990.
5. The Expert Panel: Report of the National Cholesterol Education Program Expert Panel on detection, evaluation, and treatment of high cholesterol in adults. Arch Intern Med 148:136–69, 1988.
6. Canner PL and the Coronary Drug Project Group: Mortality in Coronary Drug Project patients during a nine-year post-treatment period. J Am Coll Cardiol 8:1245–55, 1986.

7. Welsh AL and Ede M: Inositol hexanicotinate for improved nicotinic acid therapy. Int Rec Med 174:9–15, 1961.

8. El-Enein AMA, Hafez YS, Salem H, et al.: The role of nicotinic acid and inositol hexaniacinate as anticholesterolemic and antilipemic agents. Nutr Rep Int 28:899–911, 1983.

9. Sunderland GT, Belch JJF, Sturrock RD, et al.: A double blind randomised placebo controlled trial of hexopal in primary Raynaud's disease. Clin Rheumatol 7:46–9, 1988.

10. Freis ED: Rationale against the drug treatment of marginal diastolic systemic hypertension. Am J Cardiol 66:368–71, 1990.

11. Witherington R: Mechanical devices for the treatment of erectile dysfunction. Am Fam Pract 43:1611–20, 1991.

12. Susset JG, et al.: Effect of yohimbine hydrochloride on erectile impotence: A double-blind study. J Urol 141:1360–3, 1989.

13. Morales A, et al.: Is yohimbine effective in the treatment of organic impotence? Results of a controlled trial. J Urol 137:1168–72, 1987.

14. White JR, et al.: Enhanced sexual behavior in exercising men. Arch Sex Behav 19:193–209, 1990.

15. Duke JA: Handbook of Medicinal Herbs. CRC Press, Boca Raton, FL, 1985.

16. Waynberg J: Aphrodisiacs: Contribution to the clinical validation of the traditional use of *Ptychopetalum guyanna*. Presented at The First International Congress on Ethnopharmacology, Strasbourg, France, June 5–9, 1990.

17. Funfgeld EW: Rokan (*Ginkgo biloba*)—Recent Results in Pharmacology and Clinic. Springer-Verlag, New York, 1988.

18. Kleijnen J and Knipschild P: *Ginkgo biloba* for cerebral insufficiency. Br J Clin Pharmacol 34:352–8, 1992.

19. Sikora R, et al.: *Ginkgo biloba* extract in the therapy of erectile dysfunction. J Urol 141:188A, 1989.

20. Tyler VE: The New Honest Herbal. George F. Stickley, Philadelphia, 1987.

Chapter 3: Male Infertility

1. Purvis K and Christiansen E: Male infertility: Current concepts. Ann Med 24:259–72, 1992.

2. Wyngaarden JB, Smith LH, and Bennett JC (eds): Cecil Textbook of Medicine, 19th edition. Saunders, Philadelphia, 1992.

3. Carlsen E, et al.: Evidence for decreasing quality of semen during past 50 years. Br Med J 305:609–13, 1992.

4. Lauersen NH and Bouchez C: Getting Pregnant—What Couples Need to Know Right Now. Fawcett Columbine, New York, 1991.

5. Hong CY, Ku J, and Wu P: *Astragalus membranaceus* stimulates human sperm motility in vitro. Am J Chinese Med 3–4:289–94, 1992.

6. Sharpe RM and Skakkebaek NE: Are oestrogens involved in falling sperm counts and disorders of the male reproduction tract? Lancet 341:1392–5, 1993.

7. Field B, Selub M, and Hughes CL: Reproductive effects of environmental agents. Semin Rep Endocrinol 8:44–54, 1990.

8. Messina M and Messina V: Increasing the use of soyfoods and their potential role in cancer prevention. J Am Dietetic Assoc 91:836–40, 1991.

9. Aitken RJ: The role of free oxygen radicals and sperm function. Int J Androl 12:95–7, 1989.

10. Kaur S: Effect of environmental pollutants on human semen. Bull Environ Contam Toxicol 40:102–4, 1988.

11. Steeno OP and Pangkahila A: Occupational influences on male fertility and sexuality. Andrologia 16:5–22, 1984.

12. Kulikauskas VD, Blaustein D, and Ablin D: Cigarette smoking and its possible effects on sperm. Fertil Steril 44:526–8, 1985.

13. Zini A, De Lamirande E, and Gagnon C: Reactive oxygen species in semen of infertile patients: Levels of superoxide dismutase- and catalase-like activities in seminal plasma and spermatazoa. Int J Androl 16:183–8, 1993.

14. Fraga C, et al.: Ascorbic acid protects against endogenous oxidative DNA damage in human sperm. Proc Natl Acad Sci 88:11003–6, 1991.

15. National Research Council: Recommended Dietary Allowances, 10th edition. National Academy Press, Washington, DC, 1989.

16. Dawson E, Harris W, and Powell L: Effect of vitamin C supplementation on sperm quality of heavy smokers. FASEB J 5:A915, 1991.

17. Dawson EB, et al.: Effect of ascorbic acid on male fertility. Ann NY Acad Sci 498:312–23, 1987.

18. Aitkin RJ, et al.: Analysis of the relationship between defective sperm function and the generation of reactive oxygen species in cases of oligzoospermia. J Androl 10:214–20, 1989.

19. Moilanen J, Hovatta O, and Lindroth L: Vitamin E levels in seminal plasma can be elevated by oral administration of vitamin E in infertile men. Int J Androl 16:165–6, 1993.

20. Weller DP, Zaneveld JD, and Farnsworth NR: Gossypol: Pharmacology and current status as a male contraceptive. Econ Med Plant Res 1:87–112, 1985.

21. Prasad AS: Zinc in growth and development and spectrum of human zinc deficiency. J Am Coll Nutr 7:377–84, 1988.

22. Tikkiwal M, et al.: Effect of zinc administration on seminal zinc and fertility of oligospermic males. Ind J Physiol Pharmacol 31:30–4, 1987.

23. Takihara H, et al.: Zinc sulfate therapy for infertile males with or without varicocelectomy. Urology 29:638–41, 1987.

24. Netter A, et al.: Effect of zinc administration on plasma testosterone, dihydrotestosterone and sperm count. Arch Androl 7:69–73, 1981.

25. Sandler B and Faragher B: Treatment of oligospermia with vitamin B12. Infertility 7:133–8, 1984.

26. Kumamoto Y, et al.: Clinical efficacy of mecobalamin in treatment of oligospermia. Results of a double-blind comparative clinical study. Acta Urol Japan 34:1109–32, 1988.

27. Schacter A, Goldman JA, and Zukerman Z: Treatment of oligospermia with the amino acid arginine. J Urol 110:311–3, 1973.

28. Goa KL and Brogden RN: L-carnitine—A preliminary review of its pharmacokinetics, and its therapeutic use in ischemic cardiac disease and primary and secondary carnitine deficiencies in relationship to its role in fatty acid metabolism. Drugs 34:1–24, 1987.

Chapter 4: Prostate Health

1. Bosland MC: Diet and cancer of the prostate: Epidemiological and experimental evidence. In: Diet, Nutrition and Cancer: A Critical Evaluation. Reddy BS and Cohen LA (eds). CRC Press, Boca Raton, FL, 1986, pp. 125–50.

2. Oshi K, et al.: A case-control study of prostatic cancer with reference to dietary habits. Prostate 12:179–90, 1988.

3. Carter JP, et al.: Hypothesis: Dietary management may improve survival from nutritional linked cancers based on analysis of representative cases. J Am Coll Nutr 3:209–26, 1993.

4. Garnick MB: Prostate cancer: Screening, diagnosis, and management. Ann Int Med 118:804–18, 1993.

5. Hinman F: Benign Prostatic Hyperplasia. Springer-Verlag, New York, 1983.

6. Fahim M, et al.: Zinc treatment for the reduction of hyperplasia of the prostate. Fed Proc 35:361, 1976.

7. Hart JP and Cooper WL: Vitamin F in the treatment of prostatic hyperplasia. (Report Number 1.) Lee Foundation for Nutritional Research, Milwaukee, WI, 1941.

8. Scott WW: The lipids of the prostatic fluid, seminal plasma and enlarged prostate gland of man. J Urol 53:712–8, 1945.

9. DeRosa G, Corsello SM, Ruffilli MP, et al.: Prolactin secretion after beer. Lancet 2:934, 1981.

10. Judd AM, MacLeod RM, and Login IS: Zinc acutely, selectively and reversibly inhibits pituitary prolactin secretion. Brain Res 294:190–2, 1984.

11. Vescovi PP, et al.: Pyridoxine (vitamin B6) decreases opiods-induced hyperprolactinemia. Horm Metab Res 17:46–7, 1985.

12. Boccafoschi S and Annoscia S: Comparison of *Serenoa repens* extract with placebo by controlled clinical trial in patients with prostatic adenomatosis. Urologia 50:1257–68, 1983.

13. Cirillo-Marucco E, et al.: Extract of *Serenoa repens* (Permixon) in the early treatment of prostatic hypertrophy. Urologia 5:1269–77, 1983.

14. Tripodi V, et al.: Treatment of prostatic hypertrophy with *Serenoa repens* extract. Med Praxis 4:41–6, 1983.

15. Emili E, Lo Cigno M, and Petrone U: Clinical trial of a new drug for treating hypertrophy of the prostate (Permixon). Urologia 50:1042–8, 1983.

16. Greca P and Volpi R: Experience with a new drug in the medical treatment of prostatic adenoma. Urologia 52:532–5, 1985.

17. Duvia R, Radice GP, and Galdini R: Advances in the phytotherapy of prostatic hypertrophy. Med Praxis 4:143–8, 1983.

18. Tasca A, et al.: Treatment of obstructive symptomatology caused by prostatic adenoma with an extract of *Serenoa repens*. Double-blind clinical study vs. placebo. Minerva Urol Nefrol 37:87–91, 1985.

19. Crimi A and Russo A: Extract of *Serenoa repens* for the treatment of the functional disturbances of prostate hypertrophy. Med Praxis 4:47–51, 1983.

20. Champlault G, Patel JC, and Bonnard AM: A double-blind trial of an extract of the plant *Serenoa repens* in benign prostatic hyperplasia. Br J Clin Pharmacol 18:461–2, 1984.

21. Mattei FM, Capone M, and Acconcia A: *Serenoa repens* extract in the medical treatment of benign prostatic hypertrophy. Urologia 55:547–52, 1988.

22. Ask-Upmark E: Prostatitis and its treatment. Acta Med Scand 181:355–7, 1967.

23. Ohkoshi M, Kawamura N, and Nagakubo I: Clinical evaluation of Cernilton in chronic prostatitis. Jap J Clin Urol 21:73–85, 1967.

24. Buck AC, Rees RWM, and Ebeling L: Treatment of chronic prostatitis and prostadynia with pollen extract. Br J Urol 64:496–9, 1989.

25. Gallizia F and Gallizia G: Medical treatment of benign prostatic hypertrophy with a new phytotherapeutic principle. Recent Med 9:461–8, 1972.

26. Pansadoro V and Benincasa A: Prostatic hypertrophy: Results obtained with *Pygeum africanum* extract. Minerva Med 11:119–44, 1972.

27. Zurita IE, Pecorini M, and Cuzzoni G: Treatment of prostatic hypertrophy with *Pygeum africanum* extract. Rev Bras Med 41:364–6, 1984.

28. Donkervoort T, Sterling J, van Ness J, et al.: A clinical and uro-dynamic study of Tadenan in the treatment of benign prostatic hypertrophy. Urology 8:218–25, 1977.

29. Dufour B and Choquenet C: Trial controlling the effects of *Pygeum africanum* extract on the functional symptoms of prostatic adenoma. Ann Urol 18:193–5, 1984.

30. Barlet A, Albrecht J, Aubert A, et al.: Efficacy of *Pygeum africanum* extract in the medical therapy of urination disorders due to benign prostatic hyperplasia: Evaluation of objective and subjective parameters. A placebo-controlled double-blind multicenter study. Wien Klin Wochenschr 102:667–73, 1990.

31. Duvia R, Radice GP, and Galdini R: Advances in the phytotherapy of prostatic hypertrophy. Med Praxis 4:143–8, 1983.

32. Lucchetta G, Weill A, Becker N, et al.: Reactivation from the prostatic gland in cases of reduced fertility. Urol Int 39:222–4, 1984.

33. Menchini-Fabris GF, Giorgi P, Andreini F, et al.: New perspectives of treatment of prostato-vesicular pathologies with *Pygeum africanum*. Arch Int Urol 60:313–22, 1988.

34. Clavert A, Cranz C, Riffaud JP, et al.: Effects of an extract of the bark of *Pygeum africanum* on prostatic secretions in the rat and man. Ann Urol 20:341–3, 1986.

35. Carani C, Salvioli C, Scuteri A, et al.: Urological and sexual evaluation of treatment of benign prostatic disease using *Pygeum africanum* at high dose. Arch Ital Urol Nefrol Androl 63:341–5, 1991.

Chapter 5: Male Genitourinary Tract Infections

1. Purvis K and Christiansen E: Review: Infection in the male reproductive tract. Impact, diagnosis and treatment in relation to male infertility. Int J Androl 16:1–13, 1993.

2. Prodromos PN, Brusch CA, and Ceresia GC: Cranberry juice in the treatment of urinary tract infections. Southwest Med 47:17, 1968.

3. Sternlieb P: Cranberry juice in renal disease. N Engl J Med 268:57, 1963.

4. Moen DV: Observations on the effectiveness of cranberry juice in urinary infections. Wisconsin Med J 61:282, 1962.

5. Kahn DH, Panariello VA, Saeli J, et al.: Effect of cranberry juice on urine. J Am Dietetic Assoc 51:251, 1967.

6. Bodel PT, Cotran R, and Kass EH: Cranberry juice and the antibacterial action of hippuric acid. J Lab Clin Med 54:881, 1959.

7. Sobota AE: Inhibition of bacterial adherence by cranberry juice: Potential use for the treatment of urinary tract infections. J Urol 131:1013-6, 1984.

8. Ofek I, et al.: Anti-éscherichia activity of cranberry and blueberry juices. N Engl J Med 324:1599, 1991.

9. Sanchez A, et al.: Role of sugars in human neutrophilic phagocytosis. Am J Clin Nutr 26:1180-4, 1973.

10. Ringsdorf W, Cheraskin E, and Ramsay R: Sucrose, neutrophil phagocytosis and resistance to disease. Dent Surv 52:46-8, 1976.

11. Bernstein J, et al.: Depression of lymphocyte transformation following oral glucose ingestion. Am J Clin Nutr 30:613, 1977.

12. Munday PE and Savage S: Cymalon in the management of urinary tract symptoms. Genitourin Med 66:461, 1990.

13. Spooner JB: Alkalinization in the management of cystitis. J Int Med Res 12:30-4, 1984.

14. Merck Index, 10th edition, Merck & Company, Rahway, NJ, 1983, pp. 112-3, 699.

15. Frohne V: Untersuchungen zur frage der harndesifizierenden wirkungen von barentraubenblatt-extracten. Planta Medica 18:1-25, 1970.

16. Murray MT: The Healing Power of Herbs. Prima, Rocklin, CA, 1991.

17. Amin AH, Subbaiah TV, and Abbasi KM: Berberine sulfate: Antimicrobial activity, bioassay, and mode of action. Can J Microbiol 15:1067-76, 1969.

18. Johnson CC, Johnson G, and Poe CF: Toxicity of alkaloids to certain bacteria. Acta Pharmacol Toxicol 8:71-8, 1952.

19. Hahn FE and Ciak J: Berberine. Antibiotics 3:577-88, 1976.

20. Sun D, Courtney HS, and Beachey EH: Berberine sulfate blocks adherence of *Streptococcus pyogenes* to epithelial cells, fibronectin, and hexadecane. Antimicrobial Agents and Chemotherapy 32:1370-4, 1988.

21. Kumazawa Y, Itagaki A, Fukumoto M, et al.: Activation of peritoneal macrophages by berberine alkaloids in terms of induction of cytostatic activity. Int J Immunopharmacol 6:587–92, 1984.

22. Kamat SA: Clinical trial with berberine hydrochloride for the control of diarrhoea in acute gastroenteritis. J Assoc Phys India 15:525–9, 1967.

23. Desai AB, Shah KM, and Shah DM: Berberine in the treatment of diarrhoea. Ind Pediatr 8:462–5, 1971.

24. Sharma R, Joshi CK, and Goyal RK: Berberine tannate in acute diarrhea. Ind Pediatr 7:496–501, 1970.

25. Babbar OP, Chatwal VK, Ray IB, et al.: Effect of berberine chloride eye drops on clinically positive trachoma patients. Ind J Med Res 76(supp):83–8, 1982.

26. Mohan M, Pant CR, Angra SK, et al.: Berberine in trachoma. Ind J Ophthalmol 30:69–75, 1982.

27. Taussig S and Batkin S: Bromelain, the enzyme complex of pineapple (*Ananas comosus*) and its clinical application. An update. J Ethnopharmacol 22:191–203, 1988.

28. Luerti M and Vignali M: Influence of bromelain on penetration of antibiotics in uterus, salpinx and ovary. Drugs Exp Clin Res 4:45–8, 1978.

29. Tinozzi S and Venegoni A: Effect of bromelain on serum and tissue levels of amoxycillin. Drugs Exp Clin Res 4:39–44, 1978.

30. Neubauer R: A plant protease for the potentiation of and possible replacement of antibiotics. Exp Med Surg 19:143–60, 1961.

Chapter 6: Eating for Virility

1. Murray MT: The Healing Power of Foods. Prima, Rocklin, CA, 1993.

2. National Research Council: Diet and Health. Implications for Reducing Chronic Disease Risk. National Academy Press, Washington, DC, 1989.

3. Cheng KK, et al.: Pickled vegetables in the aetiology of oesophageal cancer in Hong Kong Chinese. Lancet 339:1314–8, 1992.

4. Tilvis RS and Miettinen TA: Serum plant sterols and their relation to cholesterol absorption. Am J Clin Nutr 43:92–7, 1986.

5. Messina M and Barnes S: The roles of soy products in reducing risk of cancer. J Natl Cancer Inst 83:541–6, 1991.

6. Mensink RP and Katan MB: Effect of dietary trans fatty acids on high-density and low-density lipoprotein cholesterol levels in health subjects. N Engl J Med 323:439–45, 1990.

7. Fraser GE, et al.: A possible protective effect of nut consumption on risk of coronary heart disease. Arch Intern Med 152:1416–24, 1992.

8. Sabaté J, et al.: Effect of walnuts on serum lipid levels and blood pressure in normal men. N Engl J Med 328:603–7, 1993.

9. Beynen AC, Van der Meer R, and West CE: Mechanism of casein-induced hypercholesterolemia: Primary and secondary features. Atherosclerosis 60:291–3, 1986.

10. Carrol KK: Review of clinical studies on cholesterol-lowering response to soy protein. J Am Dietetic Assoc 91:820–7, 1991.

11. Schauss A: Dietary Fish Oil Consumption and Fish Oil Supplementation. In: A Textbook of Natural Medicine. Pizzorno JE and Murray MT (eds). Bastyr College Publications, Seattle, 1991, pp. 1–7.

12. Cobias L, et al.: Lipid, lipoprotein, and hemostatic effects of fish vs fishoil ω-3 fatty acids in mildly hyperlipidemic males. Am J Clin Nutr 53:1210–6, 1991.

13. Stanto JL and Keast DR: Serum cholesterol, fat intake, and breakfast consumption in the United States adult population. J Am Coll Nutr 8:567–72, 1989.

14. Ripsin CM, et al.: Oat products and lipid lowering, a meta-analysis. JAMA 267:3317–25, 1992.

Chapter 7: Nutritional Supplements

1. Block G, et al.: Vitamin supplement use, by demographic characteristics. Am J Epidem 127:297–309, 1988.

2. National Research Council: Diet and Health. Implications for Reducing Chronic Disease Risk. National Academy Press, Washington, DC, 1989.

3. Vallee BL and Falchuk KH: The biochemical basis of zinc physiology. Physiol Rev 73:79–118, 1993.

Chapter 8: Ginseng

1. Murray MT: The Healing Power of Herbs. Prima, Rocklin, CA, 1991.

2. Shibata S, Tanaka O, Shoji J, et al.: Chemistry and pharmacology of *Panax*. Econ Med Plant Res 1:217–84, 1985.

3. Farnsworth NR, et al.: Siberian ginseng (*Eleutherococcus senticosus*): Current status as an adaptogen. Econ Med Plant Res 1:156–215, 1985.

4. Yamamoto M and Uemura T: Endocrinological and metabolic actions of *P. ginseng* principles. Proceedings of the 3rd International Ginseng Symposium, 1980, pp. 115–9.

5. Kim C, Choi H, Kim CC, et al.: Influence of ginseng on mating behavior of male rats. Am J Chinese Med 4:163–8, 1976.

6. Fahim WS, Harman JM, Clevenger TE, et al.: Effect of *Panax ginseng* on testosterone level and prostate in male rats. Arch Androl 8:261–3, 1982.

7. Hallstrom C, Fulder S, and Carruthers M: Effect of ginseng on the performance of nurses on night duty. Comp Med East West 6:277–82, 1982.

8. D'Angelo L, et al.: A double-blind, placebo controlled clinical study on the effect of a standardized ginseng extract on psychomotor performance in healthy volunteers. J Ethnopharmacol 16:15–22, 1986.

9. Yamamoto M, et al.: Serum HDL-cholesterol–increasing and fatty liver–improving action of *Panax ginseng* in high cholesterol diet-fed rats with clinical effect on hyperlipidemia in man. Am J Chinese Med 11:96–101, 1983.

10. Yun TK, et al.: A case-control study of ginseng intake and cancer. Int J Epidemiol 19:871–6, 1990.

11. Liberti LE and Marderosian AD: Evaluation of commercial ginseng products. J Pharm Sci 67:1487–9, 1978.

12. Siegel RK: Ginseng abuse syndrome. JAMA 241:1614–5, 1979.

Index